HEALING
Mushrooms

Other Books by Dr. Georges M. Halpern

L'Allergie et la Peau. Robert Laffont, Paris, France, 1976.

L'Allergia e la Pelle. Rizzoli, Milano, Italy, 1977.

Allergies. Consultations M.A., Paris, France, 1984.

Bronchial Asthma: Principles of Diagnosis and Treatment
(with M.E. Gershwin, Eds.). Humana Press, Totowa, NJ, 1993.

Ginkgo: A Practical Guide.
Avery Publishing, Garden City Park, NY, 1998.

Cordyceps: China's Healing Mushroom.
Avery Publishing, Garden City Park, NY, 1999.

Lyprinol: A Natural Solution for Arthritis and Other Inflammatory Disorders.
Avery/Penguin Putnam, New York, NY, 2001.

Lyprinol: Effective, Natural Pain Relief (in Korean).
SYS Press, Seoul Korea, 2002.

Medicinal Mushrooms: Ancient Remedies for Modern Ailments
(with A.H. Miller). M. Evans & Co., New York, NY, 2002.

The Healing Trail: Essential Oils of Madagascar.
Basic Health Books, New York, NY, 2003.

Ulcer Free!
Square One Publishers, Garden City Park, NY, 2004.

The Inflammation Revolution.
Square One Publishers, Garden City Park, NY, 2005.

Zinc-Carnosine: Nature's Safe and Effective Remedy.
Square One Publishers, Garden City Park, NY, 2005.

HEALING
Mushrooms

GEORGES M. HALPERN, MD, PhD

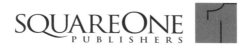

SQUAREONE
PUBLISHERS

The information and advice in this book are based on the training, personal experiences, and research of the author. Its contents are current and accurate; however, the information presented is not intended to substitute for professional medical advice. The author and the publisher urge you to consult with your physician or other qualified health-care provider prior to starting any treatment or undergoing any surgical procedure. Because there is always some risk involved, the author and publisher cannot be responsible for any adverse effects or consequences resulting from the use of any of the suggestions, preparations, or procedures described in this book.

COVER DESIGNER: Jeannie Tudor
IN-HOUSE EDITOR: John Anderson
TYPESETTER: Gary A. Rosenberg

Square One Publishers
115 Herricks Road
Garden City Park, NY 11040
(516) 535-2010 • (877) 900-BOOK
www.squareonepublishers.com

Library of Congress Cataloging-in-Publication Data

Halpern, Georges M.
  Healing mushrooms : ancient wisdom for better health /
Georges M. Halpern.
      p. cm.
  Includes bibliographical references and index.
  ISBN-13: 978-0-7570-0196-3 (pbk.)
  ISBN-10: 0-7570-0196-3 (pbk.)
  1. Mushrooms—Therapeutic use. I. Title.

RM666.M87H34 2007
615′.3296—dc22

                            2006026448

Printed in Canada

10   9   8   7   6   5   4   3   2   1

Contents

Acknowledgments

My father was a mycologist by necessity: he had to find food when he was close to starvation in Eastern Galicia during his childhood, and in Siberia during the family exile of 1916. He taught me about the *cèpes*, chanterelles, and *trompettes-de-la-mort* when we were hiding from the French police and the Gestapo in the Ardèche in 1941, and around Aiguebelette, Savoie, in 1942. It was then that I discovered the shapes, colors, the taste, and the magic of marvelous and accessible foods. During the short breaks outside the refugee camps in Switzerland (1943–1944), I found myself hoping for rain during the late summer or early fall, and would crawl back to the hidden, secret circles where these delicious mushrooms would sprout, sending their odoriferous messages to be captured only by the initiated.

My next experience with mushrooms was my initiation to the medicinal properties of *Psylocybes* during my residency as a shrink. We did not jump, fly, or get sick—we discovered a new world, shared with the *curanderas* and our schizophrenic patients. But Tomio Toda, the immunologist and Noh master, was promoting *Lentinula edodes*, the shiitake mushroom, as an immunostimulant against "our" *Corynebacterium parvum*. Soon, Lentinan, the immunomodulator made from shiitake, would be a major drug in Japan. My attraction to mushrooms was justified, and my quest would take me to the Pacific Rim, both in Asia and California.

I must thank Rudy Shur, the publisher, who is confident in the potential success of this book. Andrew H. Miller helped with an initial version of this book a number of years ago and has constantly provided interesting material. John Holliday, Ph.D., has also been of critical support and helped me in updating arcane information. Peter Weverka was the researcher and talented scribe of the first version of this book. John Anderson was the attentive, careful writer *cum* editor of this book; without his talents, this book would simply be a boring academic dissertation.

I cannot forget my wife, daughters, and grandsons, not because they escaped too often the fate of Sacha Guitry's own as described in the first pages of his *Roman d'un Tricheur,* but simply because they still love me despite the long physical and mental absences. They will need these mushrooms!

Georges Halpern, M.D., Ph.D.
Portola Valley, California

1

An Introduction to Healing Mushrooms

Mushrooms have been used as medicines by humans for 5,000 years or more. As you will see, many mushrooms have properties that can improve your health and well-being. This book presents the fascinating story of eight healing mushrooms: maitake, reishi, shiitake, *Cordyceps sinensis*, *Agaricus blazei*, *Phellinus linteus*, *Trametes versicolor*, and *Hericium erinaceus*, as well as recent findings on additional mushrooms. It explains how ancient peoples used these mushrooms and the promise they bring for healing and preventing illness in the modern world. This book presents the latest scientific and clinical research, describes the most up-to-date experiments, and conjectures about mushrooms and their power to heal.

FUNGI AND MUSHROOMS IN NATURE

What we call a "mushroom" is the fruit-body of a fungus, the reproductive part of the fungus that grows above ground and releases spores, the seed-like elements from which new fungi are made. Much as fruit is the reproductive organ of a fruit tree, a mushroom is the reproductive organ of a fungus. Typically, spores sprout from the gills, the thin brown tissue found on the underside of the mushroom cap. Borne by the wind, some kinds of spores are capable of traveling great distances from the fruit-body to start their own fungus colonies. Mushrooms produce prodigious numbers of spores. A giant puffball, for example, may produce 20 trillion: it has been calculated that if every spore from the giant puffball sprouted and grew to maturity, it would form a mass three times the size of the sun! The spores are produced in such large numbers to guarantee the spread of the fungus in the environment. Mycologist Elio Schaechter has written about spores,

"Lavishness is necessary; rare is the spore that germinates into successful fungal growth. Such wastefulness, however, is not unlike the production of millions of unsuccessful sperm cells by the human male."

Not all fungi, however, produce mushrooms. Some are able to create spores and reproduce without bearing a fruit-body. Fungi that reproduce without a sexual stage are called imperfect fungi, or *fungi imperfecti.*

In nature, fungi are the great recyclers. To feed itself, but also to assist plants in getting the nutrients they need, a fungus breaks down organic matter into essential elements. According to recent estimates by David Hawksworth, there are over 1,500,000 species of fungi on earth. Mushrooms constitute at least 14,000, and perhaps as many as 22,000, known species, but this may be less than 10% of the total. Assuming that the proportion of useful mushrooms among the undiscovered mushrooms will be only 5%, there may be thousands of as yet undiscovered species that will be of possible benefit to humankind. Even among the known species the proportion of well-investigated mushrooms is very low. About 700 species are eaten as food, and 50 or so species are poisonous.

Fungi make up about a quarter of the biomass of the earth. They need organic matter to feed on, develop, and grow; hence, they are found almost everywhere except on inlandsis, or above 25,000 feet. Strange as it may seem, seeing as they are usually associated with rot and decay, fungi are something of a cleanser in that they transform dead organic matter into nutrients that plants and animals can feed on. Without fungi, matter would not break down and decompose, and the world would be crowded with dead animals and plants.

Every fungus begins as a tiny, seedlike spore. Spores are carried by wind and water. When a spore lands in a hospitable place—a moist place that is not too hot or cold and is near a food source—it may germinate and start a new fungus colony. At that point, the spore grows hyphae, the fine, threadlike strands from which the mycelium is made. The mycelium is the feeding body of the mushroom. Composed of a latticework of interconnected hyphae threads, it is for the most part subterranean, living in soil or decayed wood, much like the root system of a plant. It can feed on almost any organic substrate: soil, wood rot, or food left for too long in the pantry.

Mushrooms are not green like many other plants because they do not contain chlorophyll, the green pigment associated with photosynthesis. In spring and summer, the most abundant substance in leaves is chlorophyll, which gives them their green color. Chlorophyll is essential for photosynthesis, the process which converts the energy of sunlight into sugar. Sunlight is also necessary for the synthesis of chlorophyll itself. During summer when the days are long and sunlight is plentiful, chlorophyll is synthesized in a steady, abundant supply, so that throughout the season the leaves remain green.

How fast and how large the mycelium grows depends on environmental factors such as soil temperature and the accessibility of food. Researchers have reported finding a mycelium beneath the soil of Michigan that is 1,500 years old and 35 acres wide, and weighs 100 tons. This mycelium is from the fungus *Armillaria bulbosa,* a root pathogen of aspen. Using molecular methods, the researchers mapped the extent of the fungus genome to show that the mycelium germinated from a single spore. (In case you're in the neighborhood, the researchers place the monster on the upper peninsula of Michigan at 45°58′28″ N, 88°21′46″ W.)

The mycelium insinuates itself into the substrate on which it feeds. It secretes complex enzymes that break down organic material in such a way that the fungus can absorb food from the substrate. Research has shown that these complex enzymes act as a growth stimulus to nearby plants. They degrade organic material so that important nutrients are returned to the soil where plants can feed on them. In this way, fungi provide the raw material for trees and plants.

Fungi are essential for a healthy forest. If there are no fungi in the soil, plants cannot grow because they cannot break down and absorb nutrients without the help of fungi. One group of mushrooms called the mycorrhizae attach themselves to the roots of trees. They act like a secondary root system, reaching deep into the soil to get nutrients that the tree could not otherwise get and passing these nutrients upward to the tree. In return, trees provide the mycorrhizal fungus with a set of nutrients that they need to grow. The fungus and tree work together in a symbiotic partnership, with some plant growth hormones produced by fungi. Many plants cannot survive without fungi.

In effect, fungi are molecular disassemblers: they take the complex compounds created by plants, such as cellulose, carbohydrates, and protein, and disassemble them so that plants can digest them. By contrast, plants are molecular assemblers, taking very simple compounds such as water, nitrogen, and carbon and combining them into complex forms such as protein, carbohydrates, and cellulose.

Some scientists believe that the ability of mushrooms to break down organic matter in nature is linked to their medicinal properties for humans. Fungi live in a hostile environment in the midst of decay at the harshest layer of the ecosystem. They encounter disease-causing pathogens far more frequently than other life-forms. To survive, they must have proactive, healthy immune functions. Some scientists believe that the antipathogenic properties developed by mushrooms as a survival mechanism are precisely what make them valuable to the human immune system.

INTELLIGENT FUNGI?

Fungi, in their own small way, may exhibit a primitive intelligence. How else can one explain advanced behavior on the part of certain fungi, such as *Cordyceps curculionum* and the amoeba-like slime mold *Physarum polycephalum*?

Cordyceps refers to different varieties of fungi that grow and feed on the bodies of insects. (Chapter 7 of this book describes *Cordyceps sinensis*, a mushroom that grows from the bodies of caterpillars in the mountains of China and Nepal.) In the case of *Cordyceps curculionum*, the spore attaches itself to an ant, germinates, begins feeding, and grows into a small mushroom. The ant, meanwhile, with the mushroom riding piggyback, goes about its normal business. One day, however, the ant is seized with a sudden desire to climb a tree, and up it goes. When it reaches a height sufficient for the release of the *Cordyceps curculionum* spores, the ant digs its mandibles into the tree and remains there for the rest of its life. When it finally dies, the spores are released from on high and are spread far and wide on the forest floor. *Cordyceps curculionum* shows admirable restraint by not eating the ant right away, a display of moderation in the presence of food that seems to demonstrate a level of intelligence.

To test the intelligence of the slime mold *Physarum polycephalum*, Toshiyuki Nakagaki of the Bio-Mimetic Control Research Center, in Nagoya, Japan, placed pieces of the mold in the middle of a five-square-inch maze. In the two exit points of the maze, he placed a food source, ground oat flakes. The idea was to see whether the fungus would abandon its normal method of foraging for food—by spreading outward from a central point of germination—and instead grow directly toward the food sources. To his surprise, Nakagaki discovered that the mold did indeed go straight toward the food sources. The organism stretched itself in a thin line along the contours of the maze until it reached the exit points. Similar to a laboratory rat, the slime mold was able to negotiate the maze and find the food.

MUSHROOMS AND THE CONNECTION TO THE EARTH

In the distant human past, all plants and animals were seen as repositories of secret power that could be used for good or ill. In a sense, the whole world was a pharmacopoeia. Our ancestors' relationship to the food they ate was very different from ours. They understood nourishment in a different way than we do: food was sacred and our ancestors believed that the plants and animals they ate were gifts from the divine. Plants and animals had spirits, and when you ate a plant or animal, you partook of its spirit as well.

In our day, most people would have trouble explaining where their food was grown or how it came to the table at which they sit. Too few people appreciate the expertise and effort that goes into cultivating and growing food. We have lost the primal connection to the food we put in our bodies and with it, we have lost our connection to the earth. Most of us understand food in terms of flavor and texture, but we don't understand that food is our connection to the earth and its vital energy.

Mushrooms are potent medicines and contain many nutrients. Mushrooms, which grow so close to the earth, have a grounding effect. When you take a medicinal mushroom, you get back in touch with the essential forces of the earth. You tap into the sustaining power that incites the animal to endeavor and the plant to grow no matter what the obstacle. Humankind has been nourished by medicinal mushrooms for many centuries. We look forward to new discoveries by which modern science will harness mushrooms' medicinal power for the good of humankind in the years to come.

LOOKING AT THE EVIDENCE

Many claims are made for medicinal mushrooms. Sometimes out of sheer enthusiasm and sometimes for commercial motives, authors make exaggerated claims. A few of these claims border on the outlandish. For example, the label on a medicinal mushroom product from China claims the following: "Effective on cancer, AIDS, hepatitis, headaches, colds, and impotence." Claims like these raise false hopes. Worse, they cause people to be cynical about medicinal mushrooms and herbal remedies in general.

For this book, I was careful to examine sources of information to make sure that they were reliable. Except for historical purposes, I have endeavored to cite only studies and experiments that were undertaken in the past five or six years in order to present the most current information about medicinal mushrooms.

Throughout this book, I present scientific studies on medicinal mushrooms, their immune-modulating capabilities, and their curative properties. Most of these studies were done in the East—in China, Korea, and

Japan. Western science has been slow to catch up to the benefits of medicinal mushrooms. Many of the studies that are now being conducted in the West were inspired by studies made in the East.

I believe that the referenced studies conducted in China, Korea, and Japan are valid, following the highest standards of scientific protocol. The methods used in the East may vary from those in the West, but the scientists uphold rigorous standards and undertake their studies in the spirit of honest inquiry. The studies I present in this book have been subjected to peer-review by panels of international scientists. Some in the West have been quick to criticize scientific data from the East, but I believe that this criticism is unwarranted.

No medicinal mushroom is a cure-all and no mushroom can make the body unassailable to disease. What mushrooms can do is stimulate the immune response, giving a powerful boost to the functions of the body that are already in place for preventing and fighting disease. Only a balanced view can convince the doubters and promote medicinal mushrooms as a means of healing the body and preventing disease.

A WORD ABOUT TAKING MEDICINAL MUSHROOMS

Finding and working with a health-care professional who understands alternative medicines may be essential if you intend to use unfamiliar treatments. Be sure to let your physician know if you are using an alternative medicine. Your physician can advise you according to your needs and also help monitor the effects of the medicine on your health. Moreover, keeping informed about the latest findings in the health field is essential for your good health.

Scientific research into medicinal mushrooms is still in its infancy. From a medical standpoint, we have only now begun to understand all the benefits of medicinal mushrooms. As more research is conducted, the studies recounted in this book will fade into footnotes. Advances in medical technology will permit research into medicinal mushrooms to go much deeper than it has now.

WHY NOT GET MUSHROOMS IN THE SUPERMARKET?

Some of the mushrooms described in this book can be purchased in gourmet markets and supermarkets. That begs the question, "Can culinary mushrooms provide the same health benefits as medicinal mushroom products?"

Culinary mushrooms are an aid to health. They appear to be a good source of B vitamins, iron, niacin, riboflavin, thiamine, and ascorbic acid. By proportion to weight, mushrooms are high in polyunsaturated fats. Cultivated varieties contain large amounts of carbohydrates and fiber. On a dry-weight basis, a mushroom is high in protein, and mushroom proteins contain essential amino acids.

The relationship between good health and a diet rich in mushrooms came to the attention of modern science when health researchers noticed that people who eat mushrooms seem to be healthier than other people. In Japan, for example, scientists discovered fewer incidences of cancer in shiitake-growing regions (shiitake is described in chapter 5). Assuming that people who lived in these regions ate the shiitake mushroom often, scientists wanted to see whether shiitake had anticancer properties. They ran many tests on shiitake and discovered lentinan, the third most widely prescribed anticancer drug in the world.

Some mushrooms are better than others. Shiitake, for example, stimulates the immune system about a hundred times more than the common white button mushroom. Maitake (described in chapter 4) does much more to aid the immune system than do morels, portobellos, chanterelles, or any other culinary mushroom. Still, all mushrooms are excellent for your health. The difference between culinary mushrooms and medicinal mushrooms is that medicinal mushrooms are a class above their culinary cousins.

Taking a mushroom product in capsule or powder form has distinct advantages because most mushroom products are made from the mycelium, the feeding body of the mushroom that grows underground. Mycelium is a potent substance, nature's way of concentrating the beneficial compounds of mushrooms. When you buy a culinary mushroom, however, you buy the fruit-body. Fruit-bodies do not always contain the potent concentrations of polysaccharides that are found in mycelium. (Mycologists are currently perfecting cultivation techniques whereby the fruit-body of mushrooms can contain potent concentrations of polysaccharides.)

What's more, medicinal mushroom products are more hygienic. The organically grown mycelium powder is sterilized before it is pressed into pills or poured into capsules. Because nonorganic, store-bought mushrooms are often sprayed with pesticides, eating them regularly may actually be harmful. For that reason, I recommend buying culinary mushrooms at special food stores and other places where organic products are sold. Taking medicinal mushrooms in pills or capsules is easier on the digestive system, too. The mycelium finds its way into the body faster than the fruit-bodies of mushrooms do.

WHAT YOU WILL FIND IN THIS BOOK

Chapter 2 looks at mushrooms in Eastern and Western cultures, and how they have been both revered and reviled throughout history. Because the use of mushrooms in traditional Chinese medicine (TCM) is mentioned throughout this book, this chapter also takes a quick look at the concepts of TCM.

As you will discover, mushrooms can make you healthy in many different ways, but they do so chiefly by awakening the immune system and making it more alert. For that reason, Chapter 3 examines the active ingredients in mushrooms and how these ingredients activate various parts of the immune system.

Following this discussion are eight chapters about healing mushrooms. Each chapter describes a mushroom's character, the history of its use as a medicine, its healing properties, its folklore, and presents the latest scientific studies conducted on that specific medicinal mushroom. In Chapter 4, you will read about maitake, a culinary mushroom that lowers cholesterol and helps against diabetes, among other things. Chapter 5 describes shiitake, the delicious culinary mushroom that many believe can help prevent AIDS. Chapter 6 is about reishi, the "mushroom of immortality," its use by ancient Taoist priests, and its antitumor and antioxidant effects.

Chapter 7 describes *Cordyceps sinensis,* the anti-aging and stamina-building mushroom that generated so many headlines in 1993 when the coach of the Chinese women's track team credited it for helping his runners break three world records in a single week. Chapter 8 concerns *Agaricus blazei,* the unusual mushroom from Brazil that many believe has the strongest antitumor activity. Chapter 9 looks at *Phellinus linteus,* a mushroom that has long been cherished in Korea as an aid against stomach ailments and arthritis. Chapter 10 examines *Trametes versicolor,* the mushroom from which Krestin, one of the world's foremost anticancer drugs, is derived. Chapter 11 delves into *Hericium erinaceus,* a mushroom that may hold promise as a cure for Alzheimer's disease. Chapter 12 deals with diverse medicinal mushrooms that have been studied only recently; some of them may well be the stars of tomorrow.

Chapter 13 takes you behind the scenes, where you discover how medicinal mushrooms are cultivated. In Chapter 14, you'll learn what to look for when shopping for healing mushroom products.

2

Mushrooms— East and West

n September 1991, hikers in the Tyrolean Alps made a remarkable discovery. On a steep, rocky ridge at 10,500 feet above sea level, they found a frozen 5,300-year-old mummy, the oldest intact human being ever discovered. The Iceman, as he came to be known, yielded much information about the Neolithic (Stone Age) period in which he lived. He carried a copper axe. Previous to the Iceman's discovery, scientists believed that humans were smelting and shaping copper 4,000, but not 5,300, years ago. Also, he may have undergone a treatment resembling acupuncture: tattoos on his legs and back were on or near the acupuncture points for treating arthritis.

To mycologists, the scientists who study fungi, the most interesting aspect of the Iceman was his medicine kit. Strung to a leather thong, he carried two walnut-sized dried fungi that researchers have identified as *Piptoporus betulinus,* a fungus known for its antibiotic properties. When ingested, it can bring on short bouts of diarrhea. Researchers determined that the Iceman suffered from intestinal parasites. He probably used the *Piptoporus betulinus* as a natural worm-killer and laxative.

If the Iceman is any proof, Neolithic Europeans used mushrooms for their medicinal qualities. Still, as this book will show, the use of medicinal mushrooms in Europe pales when compared with their use in China and Japan. Except in myth and folklore, mushrooms for medicinal purposes were nearly unknown in Western culture. Only in recent years has the West awakened to the medicinal benefits of mushrooms.

MUSHROOMS IN WESTERN CULTURE

Of all cultures, mushrooms are perhaps least valued in the West, especially in regard to their use as medicine. Egyptian hieroglyphics from 4,600 years ago show that the pharaohs believed that mushrooms were the plant of immortality. The ancient Egyptians believed that mushrooms growing in the wild were the "sons of the gods" who had been sent to earth on lightning bolts. As such, only the pharaohs were permitted to eat them.

The 16th-century missionary Bernardino de Sahagun reported that the Aztecs ate a sacred mushroom called *Teonanacatl* (*Psylocybe cyanescens* var Astoria Ossip; *Psylocybe azurescens*), which he translated to mean "flesh of the gods." In ancient China, the emperors decreed that all reishi mushrooms, which were valued as the preeminent tonic herb, be handed over to them. Why, then, have mushrooms been neglected in the West?

Until well into the Renaissance (beginning in the 14th century), Europeans looked to the ancient Greeks and Romans for their ideas about treating illnesses, and Greek and Roman physicians had little to say about the medicinal qualities of mushrooms. The Roman encyclopedist and naturalist Pliny (23–79 CE) described several types of fungi but did so inadequately—it is hard to tell which species he refers to in his writings. The first Western pharmacopoeia, *De Materia Medica,* an authority in Europe for 1,600 years, ascribes healing properties to only a single mushroom. Dioscorides (circa 40–90 CE), the author of *De Materia Medica,* offers this general description of mushrooms:

> . . . either they are edible, or they are poisonous, and come to be so on many occasions, for either they grow amongst rusty nails or rotten rags, or ye holes of serpents, or amongst trees properly bearing harmful fruits. Such as these have also a viscous concreted humor, but being laid away after they are taken up, they are quickly corrupted growing rotten. But they which are not sod in broth are sweet, yet for all that, those taken too much do hurt, being hard of digestion, choking or breeding choler.

The Roman philosopher Seneca (circa 4 BCE to 65 CE) wrote of mushrooms: "(They) are not really food, but are relished to bully the sated stomach into further eating." The French philosopher Denis Diderot (1713–1784) in his *Encyclopédie* wrote, "Whatever dressing one gives to them, to whatever sauce our apiciuses put them, they are not really good but to be sent back to the dung heap where they are born."

The aversion to mushrooms was pronounced in England and Ireland, where the inhabitants as a rule did not eat them or use them as medicine. "Most of them do suffocate and strangle the eater," wrote John Gerard in *The Herball or Generall Historie of Plants,* a compendium of the properties and folklore of plants that was published in 1597. "Treacherous gratifications," wrote John Farley about mushrooms in *The London Art of Cookery,* published in 1784.

In 1620, the English physician Tobias Venner wrote about mushrooms, "Many phantasticall people doe greatly delight to eat of the earthly excrescences called Mushrums. They are convenient for no season, age or temperament." Venner is remembered today as the author of the first tobacco warning label. "Tobacco," he wrote in *Via Recta*, "drieth the brain, dimmeth the sight, vitiateth the smell, hurteth the stomach, destroyeth the concoction, disturbeth the humors and spirits, corrupteth the breath, induceth a trembling of the limbs, exsiccateth the windpipe, lungs, and liver, annoyeth the milt, scorcheth the heart, and causeth the blood to be adjusted."

In "Mont Blanc" (written in 1816), a poem that explores the relationship between humankind and nature, Percy Bysshe Shelley paints a vivid picture of mushrooms growing on the forest floor—and he reveals the prejudices of his time and place against mushrooms:

> *And plants at whose name the verse feels loath,*
> *Fill'd the place with a monstrous undergrowth,*
> *Prickly and pulpous, and blistering, and blue,*
> *Livid, and starr'd with a lurid dew,*
> *And agarics, and fungi, with mildew and mould,*
> *Started like mist from the wet ground cold;*
> *Pale, fleshy as if the decaying dead*
> *With a spirit of growth had been animated.*
> *Their mass rotted, off them flake by flake,*
> *Till the thick stalk stuck like a murderer's stake,*
> *Where rags of loose flesh yet tremble on high,*
> *Infecting the winds that wander by.*

Not all European countries are as mycophobic as the English. In Italy, Poland, and much of Eastern Europe and Russia, mushrooms are an important part of the diet, and the first days of spring find whole families journeying to the countryside to harvest mushrooms. Generally speaking, countries that underwent rapid industrialization are more likely to be mycophobic. In those countries, where industrialization often displaced the rural population, knowledge of native mushrooms and plants is more likely to be lost. In countries with stable rural populations, mushroom lore can be handed from generation to generation as youngsters forage in the company of adults.

Almost everyone is the descendent of immigrants in the United States. For that reason, knowledge of native mushrooms cannot have been handed down in a steady line from one generation to the next. Most Americans are strangers to their mushrooms. That, more than any other reason, explains why Americans are mycophobic. The first and sometimes only thing American children learn about wild mushrooms is that some are poisonous and therefore you should never pick or eat one.

Because mushrooms usually grow in the shadows, in damp places, and in decay, and because they look strange, they were sometimes associated with demons and spirits. The strange excrescences of the forest literally appear overnight, a fantastic occurrence that could only be the work of devils. In medieval times, it was believed that thunder caused mushrooms to sprout in the forest. Many believed that devils and witches used mushrooms to cast spells.

Two prominent figures of history were killed by mushroom poisoning and their deaths may have contributed to the reputation of the mushroom as a dangerous poison. In 54 CE, the Roman emperor Claudius was poisoned by his fourth wife, Agrippina. He is supposed to have died a painful death 12 hours after eating poisonous mushrooms. The Buddha is supposed to have died by a mushroom he believed to be a delicacy. The mushroom was offered as a gift and is said to have been a type that "grew

Witches and Fungi

The ergot fungus was probably the catalyst for witch trials throughout the Middle Ages, not that the witches' accusers understood why. When the ergot fungus (*Claviceps purpurea*) invades rye and conditions are appropriately damp, peasants who eat the fungus in their rye bread may suffer from ergotism. Because wheat was highly sensitive to diseases, rot, fungal infection, and harsh weather, rye was the grain of choice among the poor masses. Bread was the principal diet in many parts of Europe during the Middle Ages, when people are supposed to have eaten a pound and a half of bread a day, making them especially susceptible to ergotism.

Ergotism causes blisters on the skin, feelings of being pricked, and burning sensations. In extreme cases, sufferers experience convulsions and have vivid hallucinations. The flow of blood to the limbs is constricted, and limbs may turn gangrenous and fall off. Some scholars blame an outbreak of ergotism for the Salem, Massachusetts, witchcraft trials of 1692. In 1943, the Swiss chemist Albert Hoffman, experimenting with ergot alkaloids, discovered the hallucinogen LSD (lysergic acid diethylamide).

underground," although nothing more is known about it. (However, some scholars believe that the Buddha died from choking on pork, not from eating a poisonous mushroom.)

The first known written reference to eating mushrooms is an epigram written by the Greek dramatist Euripedes in about 450 BCE. It tells of a woman and her three children who died from mushroom poisoning.

Mushrooms and Western Medicine

To be fair to Europeans, mushrooms may have been a part of European medicine in the past. The records are hard to come by because folk medicine was not recorded or valued during the Middle Ages in the same manner as ancient Greek and Roman medicine. What's more, Christian church officials, operating under the notion that folk healers were pagan practitioners of heathen religions, suppressed folk medicine and sometimes persecuted those who practiced it. Very little research into medicine was recorded during the Middle Ages as the monks busied themselves with copying and recopying Greek and Roman medical texts. Then, with the coming of the Renaissance, European physicians took what they believed to be a more scientific approach to their work. Folk remedies were considered backward and were shunned in favor of contemporary medicines and treatments.

All this is not to say that fungi are not used as medicine in the West. Consider these three important drugs, all of which are derived from fungi:

- Penicillin—Produced from the fungus *Penicillium notatum,* penicillin is one of the most prescribed antibiotics in the world and is routinely used to treat bacterial infections. Thanks to penicillin and other antibiotics, death rates from infectious bacterial diseases are 5% of what they were in 1900.

- Cyclosporin—Produced from *Tolypoclatium inflatum* Gams, cyclosporin A is produced by many species of filamentous Ascomycetes fungi. What is now known is that all the various fungi used, under whatever Latin name given, are all anamorphs of the species *Cordyceps subsessilus.* This drug is used in organ transplants to control the T cells of the immune system and give transplanted organs a better chance of being accepted by the body. The drug is also used as a treatment for diabetes, severe chronic urticaria with angioedema, or atopic dermatitis.

- Krestin—A polysaccharide fraction named PSK, extracted from the *Tram-*

etes versicolor mushroom, is the basis for the pharmaceutical drug Krestin. Before the advent of Taxol, Krestin was the number-one anti-cancer therapy in the world. Although not approved by the United States Food and Drug Administration (FDA), this drug has a very good track record and a loyal following among oncologists around the world.

Culinary Mushrooms

As to culinary mushrooms, the prejudice against them may be subsiding in the United States. The bland button mushroom still accounts for the majority of mushroom sales, according to the American Mushroom Institute, but sales of shiitakes, oyster mushrooms, and other more exotic culinary varieties are on the rise. Between 1989 and 1995, sales of shiitake mushrooms doubled and sales of oyster mushrooms grew by 36%. Overall, mushroom sales grew by 25%. Black and white morels, porcinis, chanterelles, portobellos, and enokis are now available in gourmet markets and some supermarkets as well. In 1999, world production of mushrooms amounted to $18 billion, roughly equal to coffee sales.

Hallucinogenic Mushrooms

In recent years, R. Gordon Wasserman, Albert Hoffman, Carl A.P. Ruck, and other scholars have proposed that ancient Greeks and Romans used hallucinogenic mushrooms in their religious rituals. Because the rituals were conducted in private and the participants were sworn to secrecy, the evidence is hard to read. But Wasserman and others make compelling arguments for the use of hallucinogenic mushrooms by Greeks, Romans, and even early Christians.

In Greek mythology, Demeter's daughter Persephone was kidnapped by Pluto, the king of the Underworld. Furious, Demeter killed all the crops, whereupon Zeus, afraid that his subjects would starve and no one would be left to make sacrifices, brokered an arrangement: Persephone would spend a third of the year in Hades with Pluto and the rest of the year above ground with her mother. The myth celebrates birth and regeneration, the return of spring, and the blessings of agriculture.

Annually, the Greeks held a festival in October to commemorate Demeter's reunion with Persephone. For several days, revelers filled the streets of Athens, and then the festival moved to nearby Eleusis, where a select few were allowed in the initiation hall. There, in the semidarkness, they drank a potion called *kykeon* ("mixture") and beheld the Mysteries of Eleusis. Initiates are supposed to have experienced convulsions and hallucinations. In a 7th-century BCE poem describing the mysteries, the poet speaks of seeing the beginning and ending of life, a vast circle starting and ending in the same place.

Kykeon was made of barley, water, and mint, and Wasserman and his colleagues believe that ergot-infested barley accounts for the hallucinogenic nature of the potion. To back up their theory, they point out that *kykeon* was purple, as is ergot sclerotia when immersed in water. Purple, the color of ergot, was also Demeter's identifying color, and an ear of grain was the symbol of the Eleusinian Mysteries.

We will probably never know for sure if drinking ergot was a feature of the Eleusinian rituals. Nevertheless, it is intriguing to think that Socrates, Plato, and other seminal thinkers of Western philosophy drank ergot, the fungus from which LSD is derived, during the festival of Eleusis.

No less a scholar than Robert Graves has suggested that followers of the Dionysos cult ate the hallucinogenic mushroom *Amanita muscaria* during their autumnal feasts. A mosaic in the ancient Christian basilica of Aquileia in northern Italy clearly shows a basket filled with *Amanita muscaria* mushrooms. Some scholars have suggested that early Christians ate the mushroom in their religious rituals, but the mosaic at Aquileia may be left over from the original Roman temple, the one from which the basilica was built.

The ritual use of the hallucinogenic mushroom *Amanita muscaria* by shamans and priests in Asia, America, and Africa is well documented. The priests of ancient Europe could have used the mushroom in their rituals, too. The Vikings are supposed to have eaten it before battle to induce the "berserk" state and make themselves more ferocious to their enemies.

The Koryak tribe of Siberia are not Europeans, but their use of *Amanita muscaria* is too interesting not to relate. Filip Johann von Strahlenberg, a Swedish explorer traveling in Siberia in the early 1700s, records how wealthy tribe members assembled in a hut to ingest the mushroom, while the tribe's poorer members, not to be denied the experience, assembled outside. When an intoxicated tribe member left the hut to urinate, those outside gathered around to collect his urine in a bowl so that they could drink and partake of the hallucinogenic mushroom, albeit secondhand.

MUSHROOMS IN THE EAST

Chinese culture is anything but mycophobic. The prejudice against fungi is entirely absent in China, and the Chinese faith in the medicinal qualities of mushrooms is unimpeachable. As anybody who has eaten in a Chinese restaurant knows, mushrooms are a feature of Chinese cuisine. Gathering mushrooms is a popular pastime in the countryside. In China's oldest materia medica, the *Herbal Classic,* many mushrooms are described, so the use of mushrooms for medicinal purposes in China reaches far into the past. (Legend has it that the *Herbal Classic* was written in the 28th century BCE by emperor Shen Nung, the Divine Plowman Emperor, but most scholars date the book to about 200 CE.)

Why are mushrooms valued in the East, but not the West, for their medicinal properties? One can only speculate on this subject, but here are a few possibilities as to why the Chinese value medicinal mushrooms so highly:

- The Chinese never drew a distinction between folk medicine and higher medicine. The physicians who compiled the *Materia Medica* included folk medicines because evidence showed that the medicines prevented disease or cured the sick. In the West, folk medicines were deemed backward and out of date, and they weren't preserved in the *Materia Medica.*

- In so far as they traded medical knowledge with one another, Buddhist monks constituted a kind of medical fraternity throughout much of Chinese and Japanese history. The monks, traveling from monastery to monastery, spread information about medicinal mushrooms.

- Taoist priests used medicinal mushrooms in their rituals and for healing purposes. Some aspects of the ancient Chinese religions, including the healing arts, are preserved in Taoism. Therefore, the Chinese never lost their connection to the past and the ways in which ancient people used mushrooms.

- China's legendary bureaucracy helped circulate information about medicinal mushrooms. Most dynasties had a medical official who was responsible for issuing and enforcing health ordinances. The provinces had their medical officials, too, who traded information with one another.

Traditional Chinese Medicine (TCM)

The traditional Chinese system of medicine represents a completely different medical language. It has been said that traditional Chinese medicine attempts to understand the body as an ecosystem or single component in nature. Where a Western doctor studies a symptom in order to determine the underlying disease, a Chinese doctor sees the symptom as part of a totality. Western medicine is concerned with isolating diseases in order to treat them. Traditional Chinese medicine seeks a "pattern of disharmony," or imbalance, in the patient.

The principles of TCM can be found in Taoism, the ancient philosophy or religion in which the practitioner strives to follow the correct path, or Tao, and thereby find a rightful place in the universe. Taoists believe that the universe is animated by an omnipresent life-energy called *Qi* (pronounced CHEE). Qi, meanwhile, comprises two primal opposites, *yin* and *yang*. The yin and yang complement each other and are always interacting. They produce change in the universe and counterbalance each other. Yin, the negative balance, represents water, quiet, substance, and night, among other things. Yang, the positive balance, represents fire, noise, function, day, and other entities. The interplay of yin and yang keeps the universe alive and vital.

In a healthy human body, Qi circulates unimpeded and the balance of yin and yang is maintained, but an excess of yin or yang or a blockage of Qi can create a pattern of disharmony and render the patient ill. No disease has a cause according to TCM. Rather, disease is a malevolent configuration of yin-yang forces in the body.

Qi flows through the body in invisible channels called meridians. In their diagnoses, acupuncturists examine the body's meridian points, the places where Qi is concentrated. If they discover that the body's Qi is congested or needs redirecting, they insert a needle in the proper meridian point.

In keeping with the Taoist idea that the body is a small-scale representation of the cosmos, much of the medical terminology is based on the workings of nature. Practitioners examine patients for dampness, wind, cold, dryness, and summer heat. As nature is organized into five primal powers (water, fire, wood, earth, and metal), the body is regulated by five organ networks (kidney, heart, spleen, liver, and lung), each with its own yin-yang energy.

Traditional Chinese medicine encompasses four different ways of treating the sick:

- Acupuncture—In acupuncture, stainless steel, gold, or silver needles are applied to the meridian points of the body. Originally, there were 365 acupuncture points, but that number has grown to 2,000 in modern times. Most acupuncturists work with 125 or so points, and a typical treatment requires inserting 10–15 needles.

- Moxibustion— Moxibustion is the application of burning substances on the meridian points of the body. Mugwort (*Artemisia vulgaris*) is usually the *moxa,* or heating substance.

- Herbal Medicine—In herbal medicine, herbs and combinations of herbs, including mushrooms, are prescribed to affect the body and bring it into balance. Medical literature describes more than 25,000 formulas (combinations of herbs) that physicians may prescribe for their patients.

- Tui Na or Acupressure—Acupressure involves the massaging and manipulating of the meridian points of the body. The massage techniques are meant to stimulate Qi energy.

Entering into the thought-system of Chinese medicine is not easy for a Westerner. The terminology can be baffling, and the system takes ideas and principles that are foreign to Western thought as its premise. To explain the success of TCM in healing the sick and preventing illness, some in the West dismiss Chinese medicine by crediting its success to the placebo effect (that belief in the efficacy of a therapy causes the healing effects). Others take the opposite tack and see traditional Chinese medicine as a sort of faith-based religion. They believe that Chinese medicine, because it is ancient and has roots in the East, is more spiritual and therefore more beneficial than Western medicine.

But traditional Chinese medicine *is* medicine. However strange it may appear to Westerners, TCM represents the culmination of 4,000 years of clinical practice and observation. Like Western medicine, TCM is an ever-evolving attempt to understand how the body works, how disease affects the body, and how to treat and prevent illness. Although the underlying philosophy is different from Western medicine, the perception of health and illness that Chinese medicine upholds is valid and true to itself.

3

The Healing Power
of Mushrooms

Mushrooms can promote good health by strengthening the immune system. They contain substances such as terpenoids and hetero-polysaccharides (amongst these are beta-glucans). The polysaccharides in mushrooms are extremely complex. There are many biologically active polysaccharides in mushrooms that are not beta-glucans, such as beta-mannans, cyclo-furans, and the alpha-bound varieties.

A word of caution: yeast-derived beta-glucans are the best source of beta-glucans, since they are cheap to produce (essentially waste yeast residue from the brewing process), but there are virtually no peer-reviewed articles in the literature showing biological effectiveness in humans for yeast beta-glucans. This is because the beta-glucans derived from *Saccharomyces cerevisiae* have extensive H-cross linking, and so take a "ball" formation rather than a "chain" formation. This makes them non-absorbable through the human gut. When one looks carefully at the references offered by the yeast beta-glucans companies, all the studies refer to mushroom species rather than to *Saccharomyces*.

Beta-glucans are a large class of molecules, and oat, yeast, and mushroom beta-glucans are quite distinct from one another. When absorbed through the intestinal membranes, they awaken the immune system and give it a boost. Mushrooms have a beneficiary effect on prebiotics in the gastrointestinal tract, helping promote healthy bacteria. They are also adaptogens, substances that help the body cope during times of stress.

MUSHROOMS AS IMMUNOREGULATORS

Problems in the immune system come in two varieties. When the immune system is underactive, it makes you susceptible to infections, cancer, and other illnesses. When it is overactive, it may create allergies and autoimmune reactions. *Autoimmune* means the immune system is overstimulated and mistakenly attacks the body. Diseases such as diabetes, lupus, and lymphoma are autoimmune diseases. AIDS, hepatitis, the flu, and colds, on the other hand, are associated with a weakened, underactive immune system.

As more research has been conducted on medicinal mushrooms, it has become evident that some of them are immunoregulators, substances that can quiet or activate the immune system, depending on the particular circumstances. An immunoregulator quiets an overactive immune system, and it increases activity when the immune system is sluggish. Basically, an immunoregulator triggers the production of white blood cells when the system is underactive, and it lowers their number when the system is overactive.

The optimal immune system is alert and ready to battle disease, but it is not overactive. An overactive immune system can cause autoimmune disorders or allergies and create trouble of its own. As immunoregulators,

The Importance of a Strong Immune System

Statistics such as these, which pertain to people in the United States, underscore the need to maintain a strong immune system:

- One of three Americans will get cancer in his or her lifetime.

- There are 1.2 million new cases of cancer each year in the United States.

- Six million Americans suffer from seasonal allergies, a disorder brought about when the immune system overreacts.

- Forty million Americans suffer from heart disease (caused initially by an inflammatory process).

- Each year, over 150,000 Americans die from infections they acquired in hospitals. Two million suffer from such infections annually (hospitals create "superbugs," and hospitalized people are weak and therefore more susceptible to disease).

- Compromised immune systems have also given rise to lasting disorders such as diabetes, asthma, eczema, inflammatory bowel disease, and Epstein-Barr viral infection. By some estimates, as much as 70% of the United States' health care budget is devoted to treating people with chronic ailments. About a third of the people who suffer from them can't go to work or attend school.

mushrooms can help the body attain optimal immune function. Mushrooms can help the immune system stay wide awake and strike the perfect balance between overactivity and sluggishness.

A BRIEF GUIDE TO THE IMMUNE SYSTEM

The immune system begins developing during the first weeks of gestation. The cell-mediated immunity that is associated with T cells develops in the womb. The fetus has an immune response very early in life. When a child is born, he or she has a fully intact natural immune response. The system is stimulated after birth (more "acquired" immunity) and reaches its peak at the onset of puberty, between ages 11 and 15 (sometimes later, if a child lives in a hygienic environment). Then, starting at age 35 or so, the immune system doesn't work as well. Some parts of the immune system are active while others are lazy, and other parts may work too well and perhaps cause autoimmune disorders. After age 50, the immune system experiences a decline. To be blunt, the human body is not supposed to live past that age. Nature, cruel and pitiless, wants you to make room for subsequent generations after your fiftieth birthday. However, advances in medical science, agriculture, and social organization have pushed life expectancies past age 75 in some countries.

In the course of a single day, the body may encounter billions of bacteria, microbes, viruses, parasites, and toxins. When you get a cut or an insect bite, bacteria and viruses enter your body. When you draw a breath, bacteria and viruses enter your lungs. When you take a bite of food, millions of germs enter your digestive tract. How the immune system handles these invaders is extremely complex and there is much that we don't know. The immune system's network of organs, cells, and molecules reaches into almost every part of the body.

One way to grasp the workings of the immune system is to think of the immune system as defending a country. The immune system has border guards, whose duty is to provide protection from outsiders. It has customs officials who check incoming cells and microorganisms to determine whether they should be admitted. If an unwanted invader penetrates the border, the immune system can mount a counterattack with its army of white blood cells. The immune system's intelligence agency keeps dossiers on undesirable bacteria and viruses so it can recognize and destroy those elements when they arrive. It also has mechanisms for handling civil wars and rebellions. If the immune system is overstimulated, it can harm the body but the system's civil guards can quiet revolts and maintain the peace. All these agencies work together to make sure that the immune system is a healthy, well-functioning entity.

The central duty of the immune system is to distinguish between what belongs to the body and what doesn't belong. For this reason, every cell that originates in the body has distinctive molecules—identification papers, so to speak—that mark it as belonging. Immune system cells normally do not attack cells that have their papers in order. However, all cells (and by-products) that originate outside the body are suspect. Foreign cells have distinctive molecules called epitopes. When the immune system encounters a

Cells of the Immune System

Medicinal mushrooms work by enhancing the activity of the immune system. Here are some of the major players in the body's immune response to infection and disease.

• **T cells**—One kind of T cell, the helper T cell, identifies invader cells with a chemical marker so that they can be destroyed by other cells. Another kind of T cell, called the cytotoxic T cell, destroys cells that have been infected by viruses or mutated by cancer. Still other T cells suppress the hyperactivity of the immune system when it gets overstimulated.

• **Cytokines**—Cytokines are messengers that alert the immune system to the presence of an invader. T cells, B cells, and macrophages secrete cytokines.

• **Natural killer cells**—Natural killer cells travel in the bloodstream looking for foreign cells. When they find a foreign invader cell, they destroy it.

• **B cells**—These cells secrete antibodies, which bind to and destroy antigens. There are many clones of B cells and each is programmed to produce a specific antibody that attacks a particular antigen.

• **Antibodies**—Each type of antibody is programmed to bind to and possibly neutralize a certain kind of antigen. Antibodies are secreted by B cells. When a B cell encounters an antigen with which it is familiar, it helps produce large plasma cells, and these cells, in turn, produce antibodies in large numbers. The antibodies go out and bind to the antigen. In effect, the B cell makes the prototype antibody for attaching to an antigen, and the plasma cell takes the prototype and creates many antibodies from it. Antibodies are members of a family of foreign cell that it recognizes and knows to be harmful, it takes steps to halt the invader. These invaders are known as antigens, which can be a bacterium, virus, microbe, parasite, or toxin. An antigen is any substance that provokes the immune system to act. The ability of the immune system to distinguish between cells that belong to the body and cells that don't belong to the body is called self-recognition.

Like the nervous system, the immune system can build a memory. When T cells and B cells are activated to fight a disease, some become memory cells that store information about the disease and pass it on to the next generation of cells. In this way, the immune system can recognize bacteria

large protein molecules called immunoglobulins. There are nine types of immunoglobulins. Some serve to help other cells in the immune system kill microorganisms, others activate cells of the immune system such as B cells, and some kill bacteria.

- **Phagocytes (monocytes, neutrophils, and macrophages)**—These are white blood cells that can engulf and destroy invaders. Monocytes circulate in the blood, macrophages circulate in the tissues, and neutrophils are found in the blood but can move into the tissues if needed.

The macrophage, a particularly powerful cell, deserves special attention because it plays an important role in boosting the immune system. Macrophages were discovered in the 1880s by Dr. Elie Metchnikoff, a Russian biologist. Noting their size and ability to devour other cells, he created the term *macrophage* from the Greek word *macro,* which means "big," and *phage,* which means "eater." Metchnikoff used the term *phagocytosis* to describe the process by which the macrophage destroys the foreign invader.

As soon as a macrophage encounters a foreign organism or substance, it engulfs and destroys it with a barrage of cell-killing enzymes. Macrophages, along with other cells such as dendritic cells, are antigen-presenting and antigen-processing cells (APCs). These cells present a harmless fraction of the antigen they have just destroyed to T cells so that T cells can learn what the antigen is and be able to recognize and attack it themselves. Next, the macrophage secretes cytokines, the cell messengers that alert the immune system to the presence of an invader. The result is a "chemical frenzy" or "immune cascade" in which natural killer cells and T cells are produced in large numbers to repel invaders. So, besides killing antigens on its own, a macrophage plays a key role in alerting the body to an attack.

and viruses it has confronted before and stop them. Throughout our lives, the immune system adds to its memory and becomes more competent at fighting disease.

The lymphatic system comprises a network of lymph nodes whose purpose is to filter out and drain contaminants and bacterial infections from the body. There are about 600 lymph nodes, or glands, most of them clustered around the neck, groin, and armpits. The system carries lymph, a fluid composed chiefly of white blood cells called lymphocytes, from the tissues to the bloodstream. As lymph flows through the body, it filters the body of disease. During an examination, doctors often feel the lymph nodes in the neck to see if they are swollen. Swollen lymph nodes mean that the nodes are producing additional white blood cells because the body is fighting an infection.

THE ACTIVE INGREDIENTS IN MUSHROOMS

Mushrooms and plants are composed of polysaccharides, which are long-chain molecules constructed from sugar units (*poly* means "many," *saccharide* means "sugar"). How the polysaccharides arrange themselves into structural units and how they bind together determine what compounds they form. For example, cellulose, the cell wall material in plants, represents a particular configuration of polysaccharides. Chitin, the cell wall material in mushrooms (as well as insects, shrimp, and sponges), represents a different configuration.

Polysaccharides present the highest capacity for carrying biological information since they have the greatest potential for structural variability. The amino acids in proteins and the nucleotides in nucleic acids can interconnect in only one way, while the monosaccharide units in polysaccharides can interconnect at several points to form a wide variety of structures. As a consequence, this variability in polysaccharide structure allows for the flexibility necessary for precise regulatory mechanisms to affect cell-cell interactions in the human body.

For example, many, if not all, Basidiomycete mushrooms (but not necessarily yeasts) have been shown to contain biologically active antitumor and immunostimulative polysaccharides. A recent review listed 650 species of Basidiomycetes that contain pharmacologically active polysaccharides that can be derived from fruit-bodies, mycelium, and culture broths.

Beta-glucan molecules (or B-glucans) are one configuration of polysaccharide. As you will see, beta-glucans are found in abundance in mushrooms and are one reason why they strengthen the immune system. The term *beta-glucan* refers to the way that the sugar units are attached to one another in the polysaccharide chain. Each glucose molecule has six carbons, and the linkage between the different carbons can occur at any position. A polysaccharide in which the molecule at the first position is linked to the next molecule at the third position is called a 1-3 beta-glucan. Most beta-glucans in mushrooms are of the 1-3 variety and known to boost the immune system. Plants, by contrast, mostly contain 1-4 beta-glucans.

A beta-glucan is a huge molecule. To see how large, consider penicillin, which has a molecular weight of 500 or more. Compounds found in plants can sometimes reach 45,000 or 50,000 molecular weight. The beta-glucan molecules found in mushrooms, however, are typically 1.5 to 2 million molecular weight. The size of mushroom beta-glucans has a lot to do with their value as immune-system stimulators, although the size and complexity of beta-glucan molecules also make it hard for scientists to study precisely why they are so beneficial to the immune system.

Medicinal mushrooms offer more than just beta-glucans. Mushrooms contain amino acids such as lysine and tryptophan, as well as nicotinic acid, riboflavin (vitamin B2), pantothenic acid, and vitamins B, C, and K. In addition, medicinal mushrooms contain terpenes and steroids, some of which have demonstrated antibacterial and antiviral activity. They are one of the few organic sources of the element germanium, which increases oxygen efficiency, counteracts the effects of pollutants, and increases resistance to diseases.

HOW BETA-GLUCANS AID THE IMMUNE SYSTEM

Beta-glucans do not in and of themselves cure disease. Rather, they help the immune system work better so that diseases can be prevented from attacking the body. Recent studies help us understand how beta-glucans stimulate the immune system: beta-glucans from fungi bind to specific membrane receptors of phagocytic cells and natural killer (NK) cells, stimulating their germ-killing abilities.

It also appears that beta-glucan molecules resemble the molecules found on bacterial cell walls. In effect, beta-glucans molecules make the body believe it is being invaded by a bacterium. When macrophages (white blood cells that guard the body against disease) encounter a beta-glucan, they believe that they have encountered a bacterium and they attack. This gives a boost to the entire immune system. Immune cells, such as T cells, are stimulated, and levels of antibodies increase. The immune system believes it is under attack and it goes into a state of high alert.

The unique molecular shape of beta-glucans permits them to bind to certain receptor cells on the surface of macrophages and other kinds of white blood cells. In effect, the beta-glucan molecule puts its key into the macrophage and unlocks it. As a result, free radicals are produced. Free radicals (molecules that have one or more one unpaired electron) help kill bacteria, viruses, parasites, and malignant cells, although they can also damage normal cells and their production must be controlled.

Within macrophages, beta-glucans have also been shown to stimulate the production of cytokines, the cell messengers that tell the immune system when it is being attacked. Cytokines aid macrophages in stopping the growth of and destroying tumors.

To test the health benefits of beta-glucans, scientists at the laboratories of Alpha-Beta Technology in Worcester, Massachusetts, incubated beta-glucans in blood and examined the results. They discovered that beta-glucans indeed caused free radicals to appear in white blood cells. Beta-glucans also stimulated the growth of megakaryocytes and myeloid progenitor cells, which develop into platelets, blood, and immune cells.

These polysaccharides, mostly beta-glucans, are biological response modifiers that activate immunological responses. Because of this capability, they accomplish the following:

• They place no additional stress on the body and cause no harm.

• They help the body to adapt to various biological and environmental stresses.

• They have nonspecific action on the body, supporting some or all of the major systems, including hormonal, nervous, and immune systems, as well as regulatory functions.

• They have weak antigenicity and minimal, if any, side effects.

Each mushroom appears to produce its own slightly different type of beta-glucan. For that reason, each mushroom stimulates the immune system in a slightly different way. As scientists focus their attention on the immune-enhancing properties of beta-glucans, we are sure to learn more about the different varieties and how they prevent disease. For example, we know that the beta-glucans from the maitake mushroom stimulate the production of T cells. *Agaricus blazei*, on the other hand, offers almost no T-cell effects but it stimulates the production of natural killer cells.

The United States Food and Drug Administration (FDA) has granted GRAS (Generally Recognized as Safe) status to beta-glucans. They can be extracted from other substances besides mushrooms, notably from algae, oats, wheat, and brewer's yeast, but mushrooms offer the greatest variety of beta-glucans.

Beta-glucan Studies

Interest in beta-glucans as a health supplement began in the 1940s, when scientists extracted a crude substance they called Zymosan from the cell walls of yeast. The researchers understood that the substance activated the immune system, but they didn't know how or why. In the 1960s, Nicholas DiLuzio of Tulane University succeeded in isolating 1-3 beta-glucan as the active component of Zymosan. Wrote Dr. DiLuzio, "The broad spectrum on immunopharmacological activities of glucan includes not only the modification of certain bacterial, fungal, viral, and parasitic infections, but also inhibition of tumor growth."

In the 1980s, Dr. Joyce Czop of Harvard University unraveled the mystery of how beta-glucans stimulate immunity. She observed a 1-3 beta-glucan docking to receptor sites on the surface of a macrophage cell and determined that this docking activity stimulated the macrophage to action. She wrote, "Beta-glucans are pharmacologic agents that rapidly enhance the host resistance to a variety of biologic insults through mechanisms involving macrophage activation."

One of the first clinical experiments with beta-glucan occurred in 1975, when Dr. Peter Mansell of the National Cancer Institute attempted to see whether beta-glucan could aid in the treatment of malignant melanoma, a dangerous form of skin cancer. Dr. Mansell injected beta-glucan into the nodules of the skin cancer in nine patients. He noted that the cancer lesions were "strikingly reduced in as short a period as five days" and, in some regions, "resolution was complete."

Interestingly, one of the first large-scale tests of beta-glucan was conducted on fish. In the 1980s, the Norwegian salmon-farming industry was hit with huge losses due to bacterial infections in the fish. The salmon were fed antibiotics, but the bacteria soon produced resistant strains and the antibiotics proved ineffective. Dr. Jan Raa, of the University of Norway, decided to try a novel technique: he introduced beta-glucans into the food supply of the fish, and the infections soon disappeared.

Over the past two decades, the number of scientific studies on beta-glucans has been growing steadily. Here are a handful of revealing trials and
studies on the immune-enhancing effects of beta-glucans:

- In a double-blind, placebo-controlled clinical trial conducted by Dr.
  William Browder of Tulane University, 21 patients who had undergone
  high-risk gastrointestinal surgery were given beta-glucan intravenously
  each day for a week. Dr. Browder and his colleagues wanted to find out
  if beta-glucan could boost the patients' immune system and reduce postoperative infections. Only 9% of the patients who received beta-glucan
  contracted infections, a figure considerably lower than the 49% in
  patients who did not receive beta-glucan. What's more, the mortality rate
  among those who received beta-glucan was zero, whereas the other
  patients who had undergone surgery for physical trauma suffered a 29%
  mortality rate.

- Scientists at Tulane University School of Medicine injected beta-glucan
  directly into the chest-wall malignant ulcers of women who had received
  mastectomies and radiation from breast cancer. The ulcer sores healed
  completely.

- In a study undertaken at Zhejiang University in Hangzhou, China, a
  beta-glucan concentrate derived from maitake mushrooms was administered to lung cancer patients who had undergone chemotherapy.
  Patients who received the concentrate as well as the chemotherapy had
  higher survival rates than patients who received only the chemotherapy.

- To test the effect of beta-glucan on fungal infections, scientists at the State
  University of São Paulo, in Brazil, gave conventional antifungal drugs to
  two test groups, with one group also receiving beta-glucan intravenously for one month. Thereafter, the group was given monthly doses for 11
  months. At the end of a year, the group that had received beta-glucan did
  not have a single relapse, whereas the other group experienced five
  relapses in just eight patients. Members of the beta-glucan group also
  had lower traces of fungal infection in their blood.

Beta-glucans and Cholesterol

Beta-glucans have a demonstrated ability to lower cholesterol levels. The
United States Department of Agriculture (USDA) conducted a study to
determine if adding beta-glucans to the diet lowers cholesterol levels.
Twenty-three volunteers suffering from high cholesterol took part in the

study. In the first week, all were put on a diet in which 0.8% of their calories came from beta-glucans and 35% came from fat. Starting in the second week, one group of volunteers received an oat extract with 1% beta-glucan, and another group received an oat extract with 10% beta-glucan. After three weeks, when the study concluded, cholesterol levels in the group that received the larger amount of beta-glucans dropped significantly. Cholesterol levels dropped in the other group as well, but not as dramatically. Researchers are not certain why beta-glucans lower cholesterol levels. One theory is that beta-glucans trap bile acids, which were made from cholesterol, and flushes them from the body. As bile acids leave the body, cholesterol does too. Another theory is that beta-glucans decrease the production of cholesterol by the liver.

Beta-glucans and Asthma

Asthma is a chronic inflammatory disorder that causes the small airways in the lungs to narrow. The narrowing can be triggered by pollutants, smoke, pollen, dust, or other stimuli. Five percent of the population of the United States suffers from asthma. Interestingly, asthma rates are higher in industrialized countries than developing countries. Some physicians believe that the high rates of asthma in industrialized countries are caused by the relative cleanliness of those countries. These physicians believe that the body, especially in childhood, needs to be exposed to mycobacteria, viruses, and parasites so that it can learn to fight off microbes, the so-called "hygiene hypothesis." People in developing countries, these physicians argue, do not contract asthma as often because their bodies have learned to counteract mycobacteria.

One theory is that beta-glucans can help prevent asthma because beta-glucan molecules are similar in shape to those of mycobacteria. The theory is that asthma sufferers and people who are susceptible to asthma can use beta-glucans as a substitute for mycobacteria. In so doing, they can build up the T-cell response that could help prevent asthma.

Absence of Beta-glucans in the Modern Diet

As we have demonstrated, 1-3 beta-glucans help the body build a strong immune system. Beta-glucans stimulate the production and activity of T cells, natural killer cells, and macrophages. Some scientists believe that cancer, arthritis, allergies, and other diseases that result from a weakened immune system are on the rise because people are not getting enough 1-3 beta-glucans in their diet. Processed and fast foods are probably to blame.

As explained earlier, plants contain mostly 1-4 beta-glucans, but plants contain a small amount of 1-3 beta-glucans—the kind found in mushrooms—as well. Oats and wheat have the highest 1-3 beta-glucan levels. In these grains, as much as 2%–3% of the molecules are 1-3 beta-glucans. In the past, most people obtained their 1-3 beta-glucans from grains such as oats and wheat, but the amount of 1-3 beta-glucans in those grains has dropped in recent years. Modern food-processing companies prefer grains with low 1-3 beta-glucan levels: these grains contain less fiber and they are easier for people to digest. Animals who eat corn and oats with low levels of 1-3 beta-glucans absorb the grains better and do not produce as much dung (a useless byproduct on the modern farm, where chemical instead of natural fertilizers are used). In beer production, 1-3 beta-glucan is undesirable because it confers cloudiness to the beer. Therefore, commercial strains of barley with low 1-3 beta-glucan content have been developed, primarily for the brewing industry.

Because modern food-processing companies prefer grains with less fiber (and less 1-3 beta-glucans), farmers grow those grains. The result is a loss of 1-3 beta-glucans in the modern diet, a loss for which you can compensate by making medicinal mushrooms a part of your diet. Much of the active polysaccharides, water soluble or insoluble, isolated from mushrooms, can be classified as dietary fibers (i.e., beta-glucan, xyloglucan, heteroglucan, chitinous substance) and their protein complexes. Many of these compounds have carcinostatic activity and will absorb possible carcinogenic substances and hasten their excretion from the intestines. Thus, mushrooms in general may have an important preventative action for colorectal carcinoma.

ANTI-INFECTIOUS TERPENOIDS IN MUSHROOMS

Many medicinal mushrooms contain terpenoids, which are anti-infectious agents. Terpenoids help the immune system and the healing process in various ways. Generally speaking, they are good at killing bacteria and viruses. Some terpenoids protect the arteries of the heart, and many of them are anti-inflammatory. This means that they prevent the immune system from overreacting.

The word *terpenoid* comes from the same root as "turp" in *turpentine*. Turpentine, made from the resin of pine trees, has been used as an antiseptic since the time of the ancient Greeks. Terpenoids are found throughout

nature, not just in turpentine. Like turpentine, many substances and plants that contain terpenoids give off a slightly bitter aromatic odor.

The anti-inflammatory role of terpenoids is especially valuable to the healing process. To see why, consider what happens when you get a cold. The cold virus causes the nose and throat to swell and redness to appear around the nostrils and nose. The swelling and the redness are part of the inflammatory process due to reactions of the immune system. The immune system sends white blood cells to attack the infection, and as more white blood cells arrive, the area around the infection starts swelling. Sometimes, however, there is too much swelling and an inflammatory reaction occurs. In the case of a cold, the inflammatory process exceeds it goal and the nose and throat constrict and breathing becomes difficult.

An inflammatory reaction in the arteries can have especially bad consequences. In this case, the wall of the artery can swell and encumber the flow of blood. Many physicians believe that heart disease is caused initially by an inflammatory reaction in the arteries. This is why many doctors recommend aspirin to patients. Aspirin, like the terpenoids, is anti-inflammatory. The inflammation that accompanies an infection is healthy as long as it is kept under control. To control inflammation, if necessary, we can use anti-inflammatory substances, but many of these substances also block the benefits of the immune response. Cortisone, for example, prevents inflammation but also allows germs to proliferate.

The beauty of terpenoids is that they temper the action of the immune system's response to infections—they are anti-inflammatory—but not to the extent that they prevent the white blood cells from doing their job. They stimulate the body's immune defenses, kill germs, prevent inflammation, and provide a degree of comfort. By the way, terpenoids are some of the oldest medications. To cure the common cold, people have been inhaling the fresh resin of pine trees and eucalyptus leaves for many years. Pine tree resin and eucalyptus leaves both contain terpenoids.

MUSHROOMS AS ADAPTOGENS

The term *adaptogen* was coined in the 1940s by a scientist of the defunct Soviet Union named Dr. Nicolai Lazerev. In his studies of wild Siberian ginseng, Dr. Lazerev noticed that the herb had a quieting effect on the nervous system and helped reduce the effects of stress on the body. Dr. Lazerev used the term *adaptogen* to describe herbs like ginseng that help the body adapt during times of stress. Two colleagues of Dr. Lazerev, I.I. Brekhman and I.V.

Dardymov, refined the definition of an adaptogen as follows: "[It] must be innocuous and cause minimal disorders in the physiological functions of an organism, it must have a nonspecific action, and it usually has a normalizing action irrespective of the direction of the pathological state." In traditional Chinese medicine, adaptogenic herbs and medicines are usually called tonics. A tonic herb is one that makes the body more resilient and strengthens the body's natural defenses.

Scientists are discovering that stress engages many different areas of the body: the nervous system, the cardiovascular system, hormone production, and others. The problem, some scientists believe, is that the body's response to stress was conditioned in prehistoric times when humankind faced acute, short-term, life-threatening stress, not the long-term, persistent stress and anxiety we face today. When the body experiences stress, the adrenal glands secrete hormones, the sympathetic nervous system quickly arouses itself, the heart beats faster, blood pressure rises, and the amount of sugar in the blood increases.

Some scientists believe that the body often overreacts to stress. Sustained periods of stress can tax the nervous system and cardiovascular system and disrupt hormone production. Long-term stress can lead to cardiovascular disease, fatigue, and depression. The cumulative effect of all this may result in a weakened immune system.

For example, to help cope with stress, the adrenal glands produce increased amounts of a hormone called cortisol. Increases in cortisol are normal when faced with a life-threatening situation: the adrenal glands secrete higher levels of cortisol to reduce unnecessary and painful inflammation and thereby heal wounds. However, long-term increased levels of cortisol can cause diabetes and fatigue, as well as weaken the immune system. Adaptogens are believed to let the adrenal glands recharge, stabilize the body's hormone production, and help the body control blood sugar levels. Many herbs are considered to have adaptogenic properties, including different varieties of ginseng, astragalus, and licorice root. Three mushrooms described in this book—maitake, shiitake, and reishi—are considered adaptogens.

MUSHROOMS AS PREBIOTICS

You may be interested to know that there are 10,000 times more germs in your gastrointestinal tract than there are cells in your body. By some estimates, bacteria in the large intestine account for 95% of all cells in the body.

Most people carry around 3–4 pounds of bacteria in their gastrointestinal tract. These germs amount to an ecosystem that is different in the body of each individual. Some of the bacteria are good and some may be bad. *Bifidobacteria*, for example, prevent diarrhea and constipation. Pathogenic *E. coli*, on the other hand, causes severe cramps, diarrhea, and sometimes death. Due to diet, viral and bacterial infections, or the use of antibiotics, normal bacteria in the intestinal tract can be depleted. When this happens, pathogenic bacteria may predominate and cause an illness.

Prebiotics are substances that help the good bacteria in the intestinal tract. They are a sort of intestinal fertilizer in that they promote the growth of beneficial bacteria and they control microorganisms that are not helpful. They also produce vitamins of the B family, assist the body in absorbing minerals such as calcium and magnesium, and aid the immune system by killing pathogens. Some researchers believe that they also lower blood cholesterol, prevent diarrhea, and help fend off colon cancer.

High-fiber foods such as mushrooms are prebiotics. These foods help bacteria in the large intestine to breed in a balanced, harmonious way. Mushrooms are a class above many other prebiotics because they contain terpenoids that are antimicrobial but don't affect the good germs in the intestinal tract. Mushrooms also stimulate M cells in the lining of the intestine, similar to antigen-presenting cells, which control antigens and microbes and also pass along samples of the antigens and microbes they have helped destroy to the immune system. In this way, the immune system is informed, instructed, awakened, and put on alert for invaders.

By the way, be careful not to confuse prebiotics with probiotics. A probiotic is a live bacterial culture like that found in yogurt and other fermented dairy products. Probiotics are also good for the intestinal tract, providing bacteria that the intestinal tract needs to stay healthy.

MUSHROOMS AS ANTIOXIDANTS

A free radical is an atom of oxygen whose composition is the same as that of bleach. As everyone knows, bleach is used in the household to kill bacteria, and it is used the same way in the body. To kill bacteria, viruses, parasites, and malignant cells, white blood cells and macrophages release free radicals. However, if these cells proliferate too freely, they may also kill normal cells. As a result, body tissue dies and the body ages faster.

Substances called antioxidants are capable to a certain extent of reversing the damage that free radicals do to body tissues. Perhaps the three most well-known antioxidants are vitamin C, vitamin E, and beta-carotene. Taking antioxidants helps reduce unnecessary free radicals. By bringing the number of free radicals to a normal, more acceptable level, antioxidants control the aging process. Mushrooms are also antioxidants. The good news for people who make mushrooms a part of their diet is that they never run the risk of stimulating the unnecessary production of free radicals. Mushrooms do not produce excess free radicals anywhere in the body.

PROTECTIVE EFFECT ON THE LIVER

The liver is the body's second largest organ (the skin is its largest) and one of its job is to detoxify the body. The liver is also the body's chemical plant: it manufactures cholesterol, which every membrane of every cell needs. The liver produces approximately 20 proteins, including antibodies and the proteins that are involved in the inflammatory process by which the immune system attacks infections. These proteins ensure that the body fights infections without going to excessive lengths. If the liver doesn't function well, the inflammatory process is impaired.

It appears that some substances in mushrooms have a protective effect on the liver. Mushrooms have been used to treat a variety of liver disorders, including hepatitis, a disease that infects 350 million people worldwide, according to the World Heath Organization. In a study of 355 cases of hepatitis B treated with the Wulingdan pill, which includes the fruit-body of the reishi mushroom, 92% of the subjects showed positive results. Lentinan, the drug derived from *Lentinula edodes* (the shiitake mushroom), has shown favorable results in treating chronic persistent hepatitis and viral hepatitis B. *Trametes versicolor* is sometimes prescribed for chronic active hepatitis and hepatitis B.

4

Maitake

*M*aitake means "dancing mushroom" in Japanese (*mai* means "dance"; *take* means "mushroom"). How the mushroom got its name depends on which story you choose to believe. In one account, the mushroom got its name because people danced with joy upon finding maitake mushrooms in the forest. They may well have danced with joy during Japan's feudal era, when local lords paid tribute to the shogun by presenting him with maitake mushrooms, among other gifts. To obtain the maitake mushrooms, the local lords are supposed to have offered anyone who found one the mushroom's weight in silver, a cause for dancing indeed. Another story says that the dancing mushroom got its name because the overlapping fruit-bodies give the appearance of a cloud of dancing butterflies.

In the English-speaking world, maitake is known as "Hen of the Woods." The mushroom, growing as it does in clusters, is said to resemble the fluffed tail feathers of a brooding hen. Less frequently, the mushroom is called "Sheep's Head." It is sometimes called the "king of mushrooms" on account of its size. The mushroom's Latin name is *Grifola frondosa*. *Grifola* is the name of a fungus found in Italy. Some scholars believe that the fungus got its name from the griffin (or griffon), the mythological beast with the head and wings of an eagle and the hind legs and tail of a lion. *Frondosa* means "leaflike," as the overlapping caps of maitake mushrooms growing in the wild give the appearance of leaves.

MAITAKE IN THE WILD

The chief characteristic of the maitake mushroom is the fact that it grows in clusters. The caps, which are typically 4–5 inches across, overlap one anoth-

Maitake

Maitake is a delicious culinary mushroom but is also valued for its medicinal properties. Traditionally, maitake was used in Japan as a tonic to boost the immune system and increase vitality, and the mushroom was purported to prevent cancer and high blood pressure.

• Name: Latin name, *Grifola frondosa*: *Grifola* is the name of a fungus found in Italy; *frondosa* means "leaflike." *Maitake* means "dancing mushroom" in Japanese; also known as "Hen of the Woods" and "Sheep's Head."

• Description: Grows in clusters; the caps, which are typically 4–5 inches across, overlap to form a sort of clump. A typical maitake cluster is the size of a volleyball.

• Habitat: Maitake grows at the base of oak trees, beeches, and other dead or dying hardwoods. Favors temperate northern forests; indigenous to northeast Japan, Europe, Asia, and the eastern side of the North American continent.

• Active ingredients: Beta-glucans, fractions D and MD; Grifon-D.

• Uses: Helps control diabetes; helps lose weight; lowers HDL ("bad") cholesterol; anti-HIV; helps control high blood pressure; anti-prostate and bladder cancer; protects the liver; immunomodulator.

er to form a sort of clump. The stems, meanwhile, fuse together. Maitake grows at the base of oak trees, beeches, and other dead or dying hardwoods. According to folklore, the mushroom prefers to grow where lightning has scarred the wood of a tree. A typical maitake cluster is the size of a volleyball. Clusters can be 20 inches in diameter and weigh as much as 80 pounds. The mushroom prefers temperate northern forests. It is indigenous to northeast Japan, Europe, Asia, and the eastern side of the North American continent. Connoisseurs favor maitake mushrooms from Japan for their flavor.

Commercial techniques for the cultivation of maitake mushrooms were not perfected until the late 1970s. Before then, the only way to harvest maitake was to pick it in the wild. Foragers in Japan were said to be very covetous of the secret places where maitake grew. To mark their forest turf and keep others away, foragers cut hatch marks into trees. Known locations of maitake were called "treasure islands" and where to find them was a carefully guarded secret. Many a forager kept the secret his entire life and revealed it only in his will so that his eldest son could find his way to the treasure.

Since maitake cultivation is a recent development, only within the past two decades have producers been able to switch from a reliance on foraged maitake to offering cultivated maitake. Japanese commercial cultivation, mainly for food, started in 1981 with 325 tons. Commercial maitake production worldwide may now be in excess of 50,000 tons.

RESEARCH STUDIES ON MAITAKE

Maitake is a delicious culinary mushroom, but the Japanese also value it for its medicinal properties. Traditionally, maitake was used in Japan as a tonic to boost the immune system and increase vitality, and the mushroom was supposed to prevent cancer and high blood pressure. For that reason, researchers turned their attention to maitake's effect on those diseases when they first began experimenting with maitake three decades ago. In recent years, the maitake mushroom has become a popular subject of study. In Medline, the online database of the National Library of Medicine, there are more studies pertaining to maitake than to any other mushroom covered in this book.

In 1984, Japanese mycologist Hiroaki Nanba, of the Kobe Pharmaceutical University, identified a substance found in both the mycelia and the fruit body of maitake that had the ability to stimulate macrophages. This so-called D-fraction is a standardized form of beta-glucan polysaccharide compounds (mainly beta-D-glucan). In 1984, a patent was issued in Japan to Nanba and others. Into the 1990s, Professor Nanba and his colleague Keiko Kubo continued to study maitake, trying to improve upon the antitumor and immunopotentiating activity of the D-fraction. Further purification of the D-fraction yielded the MD-fraction, which Nanba and Kubo believe to be even more bioactive. Essentially, the D- and MD-fractions have the same beta-glucan configurations, but the MD-fraction is more purified and is orally bioavailable.

Maitake and Diabetes

Diabetes is caused by abnormally high levels of glucose, or sugar, in the blood. The disease is an autoimmune disorder in which the immune system does not function properly and works contrary to itself. Diabetes is brought about when immune cells mistakenly attack the cells in the pancreas responsible for producing insulin, the hormone in charge of converting sugar into energy. The result is a sugar buildup as the body is unable to burn off excess blood sugar. An estimated 16 million Americans have diabetes and the disease contributes to nearly 200,000 deaths annually. Symptoms include excessive thirst, frequent urination, fatigue, a tingling sensation in the hands and feet, and unexplained weight loss.

Diabetes mellitus is a disease in which nutrition and medical therapy play an important role. For example, dietary fiber (as well as other nutrients) is effective in inhibiting glucose absorption, whereas other nutrients increase insulin sensitivity. A high ratio of polyunsaturated to saturated fatty acids in the diet increases insulin sensitivity, both in animal models and in a limited number of human studies. Antioxidants have been shown to be effective as well.

To find out if maitake has any effect on diabetes, researchers in Japan fed powder from the fruit-body of the mushroom to diabetic mice. The mice received 1 gram of powder a day and researchers noticed a decrease in blood sugar in the mice. What they found most interesting about their experiment, however, was an increase in insulin production on the part of the mice. It appears that maitake can help diabetes sufferers in two different ways. Maitake increases the production of insulin and controls glucose levels as well—in mice at least, and more recently in diabetic rats.

People who have diabetes will be glad to know that most mushrooms, maitake included, appear to lower blood sugar levels. However, if you are hypoglycemic—if you have *low* blood sugar levels—you should take maitake only after consulting a physician. Taking maitake may bring your blood sugar levels even lower and cause health complications. Dizziness, fainting, sweating, headaches, and malaise are symptoms of hypoglycemia. One of maitake's major mechanisms of action is as an alpha-glucosidase inhibitor, limiting the digestion of starch and absorption of sugars. Therefore, for maximum effect in diabetics, it should be taken with meals.

Recent research has focused on enhancing maitake's properties in controlling glucose metabolism, and possibly preventing diabetes, by creating a synergistic effect between maitake and other mushroom extracts, such as *Coprinus comatus* and *Cordyceps sinensis*. Other nutrients, such as the Indian herb *Salacia oblonga*, cinnamon, biotin, and chromium picolinate, may also be added to mushroom supplements. All of these components have demonstrated activity in controlling high blood sugar, as well as anti-diabetic properties in controlled clinical studies. A multi-mushroom combination with maitake may result in better efficacy, a reduction in the number of doses, and increased tolerance.

Maitake and Cholesterol

Cholesterol is a fatty, waxlike material produced by the liver that is essential for cell renewal, hormone production, and other important bodily functions. There are two kinds of cholesterol. High-density lipoprotein (HDL or "good") cholesterol carries lipids (fat) through the blood and keeps lipids from collecting. Low-density lipoprotein (LDL or "bad") cholesterol deposits lipids in the liver and on the walls of blood vessels, where it can accumulate and cause harm. People who have a diet that is high in saturated fats run the risk of getting high cholesterol levels in their blood. High cholesterol can lead to hyperlipidemia, atherosclerosis, and other health problems.

Maitake mushrooms may have an inhibiting effect on the production of lipids, and therefore have the ability to lower cholesterol levels. Scientists at Kobe Pharmaceutical University in Japan ran experiments on two groups of mice with hyperlipidemia. Both groups were fed a high-cholesterol diet, but one group's diet was supplemented with maitake powder. The maitake-fed mice had fewer lipids in their livers *and* their blood. An interesting sidelight of the experiment was the effect of maitake on good cholesterol in the maitake-fed mice. Usually, levels of HDL cholesterol decrease under the effect of a high-cholesterol diet. In the case of the maitake-fed mice, however, HDL cholesterol levels remained the same.

The Power of Synergy

Synergy implies that nutrients or other substances taken together influence one another, often magnifying each other's effects. Synergy is a common finding with natural products and medications, although the underlying mechanisms are quite complex. The best studied example involves grapefruit juice. Grapefruit juice acts by blocking the activity of some cytochrome P-450 enzymes in the intestinal wall, thereby preventing the first-pass metabolism of a wide range of drugs and natural substances metabolized by those enzymes. Calcium channel antagonists, neuropsychiatric medications, statins, and antihistamines are just a few of the drug classes significantly affected by the consumption of grapefruit juice; foods with medicinal properties and nutraceuticals may also be affected. Foods and herbs, as well as combinations of natural supplements, often produce a stronger healing effect because of the synergistic effects of the active ingredients.

Maitake and Blood Pressure

In subjects with a tendency to low blood pressure and fainting, maitake extracts (or even gourmet dishes containing the mushroom) have been known to exacerbate this tendency. It seems natural then to use extracts of *Grifola frondosa* to control high blood pressure or hypertension, a major factor in cardiovascular disease and heart attacks. But in patients with hardened arteries, maitake was not always active enough, so research has been conducted on combinations of mushrooms to increase activity. Interesting synergistic results should be expected from a combination of maitake extract, reishi (*Ganoderma lucidum*), and *Cordyceps sinensis.* This mix of traditional mushroom extracts seems much more active, while totally safe, than maitake alone.

Maitake and HIV/AIDS

In the late 1980s, Japanese researchers determined, in a non-controlled animal trial, that oral doses of the D-fraction exhibited an enhancing effect on helper T cells, the cells targeted by HIV. This was one of the earliest clinical indications that maitake might be a potential treatment against HIV.

In 1991, a maitake fraction was found to be active in a preliminary anti-HIV drug screening test conducted by the National Cancer Institute (NCI). According to the NCI's Developmental Therapeutics Program, the maitake test compound showed significant dose-related antiviral activity. Although the maitake fraction resembled the anti-HIV potency of AZT (zidovudine, formerly azidothymidine), it was not considered a promising treatment because of potential cellular toxicity *in vivo.*

Since then, much of the research into the immunomodulating effects of MD-fraction supports its potential use against HIV. The MD-fraction was the subject of a recent long-term human study on its potential to benefit HIV-infected patients. Professor Nanba and colleagues looked at the effect of 6 g of tablets, or 20 mg of purified MD-fraction combined with 4 g of tablets per day, for 360 days on 35 HIV-positive subjects. The researchers monitored CD4+ (helper T cell) counts, viral load, symptoms of HIV infection, status of secondary disease, and subjects' sense of well-being. Effects on the helper T cell count and viral load were variable: helper T cells increased in 20 patients, decreased in 8 patients, and remained static in 4 patients. Viral load decreased in 10 patients, increased in 9 patients, and was unchanged in 2 patients. Some 85% of respondents, however, reported an increased sense of well-being with regard to symptoms and secondary diseases caused by HIV infection. The researchers concluded that the MD-fraction appeared to work on several levels: by direct inhibition of HIV, stimulation of the body's own natural defense system against HIV, and making the body less vulnerable to opportunistic disease.

Interestingly, *Grifola frondosa* D-fraction together with dimethyl sulfoxide (DMSO) has also shown success in treating AIDS-associated Kaposi sarcoma, a malignant skin tumor.

Maitake and Prostate Cancer

The problem with any malignancy, including prostate cancer, is that the malignant cells do not want to die. They want to live forever and they want to proliferate, which can be very dangerous. Recently, scientists from the Department of Urology at New York Medical College in Valhalla, New York, conducted experiments to study the effect of maitake on prostate cancer cells. The scientists isolated and grew hormone-resistant prostate cancer cells. The cells were then treated *in vitro* with a highly purified beta-glucan extract from maitake called Grifon-D. After 24 hours, the scientists examined the prostate cancer cells and discovered that almost all of them had died.

The scientists also wanted to know how the Grifon-D extract worked in combination with vitamin C. Their experiments produced an interesting result: vitamin C may make maitake more effective. By including vitamin C in the dose, the scientists were able to get the same results—death of the majority of prostate cancer cells—with one-eighth the amount of Grifon-D. Vitamin C appears to enhance the antioxidant effect of maitake (antioxidants help reverse the damage that free radicals do to body tissue). The scientists concluded that beta-glucan from maitake may have use as an alternative therapy for prostate cancer.

Maitake and Bladder Cancer

Researchers at Gunma University, in Japan, conducted an experiment to determine the inhibiting effect of different mushrooms on bladder cancer. For the experiment, laboratory mice were fed a carcinogen called BBN (known to cause cancer of the bladder) every day for eight weeks. The mice were divided into four groups. One group was given no mushroom supplement, one was given shiitake mushrooms, one maitake mushrooms, and the last group oyster mushrooms (*Pleurotus ostreatus*).

After eight weeks, the scientists examined the mice to see which had developed bladder cancer. In the group that received no mushroom supplement, 100% had contracted cancer. In the maitake group, 46.7% (7 of 15 mice) developed cancer; in the shiitake group, 52.9% (9 of 17 mice) developed cancer; and in the oyster mushroom group, 65% (13 of 20 mice) developed cancer. In terms of protection against cancer of the bladder, maitake works better than shiitake and oyster mushrooms.

The experiment also yielded interesting results concerning macrophages, the powerful immune system cells that attack foreign materials. Normally, macrophages move to their prey in much the same way that a dog comes running when it smells food. Macrophages are attracted to cells that appear to be foreign. Carcinogens such as BBN, however, suppress or numb macrophages' ability to find foreign cells quickly. This experiment, however, revealed that mushrooms actually protect macrophages from being numbed. Among mice who had received mushroom supplements in their diet, macrophages were still very active despite being exposed to the carcinogen.

The three mushrooms in the experiment had a similar effect on lymphocytes, the white blood cells that circulate in the lymph nodes and flush viruses and bacteria from the body. Lymphocyte activity in the group of mice that did not receive a mushroom supplement was impaired, but the lymphocytes in the other mice maintained a normal level of activity.

Maitake as an Adjunct to Chemotherapy

Unpublished preliminary clinical data on maitake's use as an adjunct to chemotherapy were reported in 1997 by Hiroaki Nanba. A non-randomized clinical study using maitake D-fraction was conducted with a total of 165 cancer patients in stage III–IV, from 25–65 years old. Patients were administered either tablets containing maitake D-fraction with whole powder, or the maitake tablets, along with chemotherapy. According to Dr. Nanba, "The results suggest that breast, lung, and liver cancers were improved by maitake, but it was less effective against bone and stomach cancers or leukemia." The best response rates were from combining maitake and chemotherapy. Most of the patients under the maitake treatment claimed improvement of overall symptoms, even when the tumor regression was not observed. Some of the chemotherapy side effects, such as lost appetite, vomiting, nausea, hair loss, and pain, were ameliorated.

Maitake and Obesity

Maintaining the right body weight is important for your health. According to the United States Centers for Disease Control (CDC), obesity (defined as being 30% or more above ideal body weight) increased from 12% of the population in 1991 to 17.9% in 1998. Why are many people obese? Some genes are associated with obesity, and environmental factors also come into play. In the United States, time spent in front of the television can genuinely be considered a cause of obesity. TV broadcasts messages that encourage people to eat fast food, foods of dubious nutritional value, and foods loaded with "empty" calories. Television watchers are sedentary. Between eating the fast food that the TV encourages them to eat and the idle time they spend in front of the television, viewers are prone to gain weight.

Recently, scientists at Mukogawa Women's University, in Nishihomiya, Japan, wanted to see what effect maitake had on the C3H10T^1/$_2$B2C1 cell. This cell is normal in most aspects, but it has the potential to balloon and turn into an *adipocyte,* a kind of fat cell. You could say that these cells have the potential to become obese. For that reason, observing this kind of cell is useful for determining how substances affect weight loss and gain. The result of the experiment showed that maitake inhibits the conversion of normal C3H10T^1/$_2$B2C1 cells into adipocytes.

Animal studies have shown that maitake, as a major component of the diet, can inhibit weight gain. When rats were fed dried maitake powder as 20% (by weight) of a high-cholesterol diet, it significantly inhibited increases in body weight and body fat. A similar protocol promoted improved fat metabolism among maitake-fed rats, which weighed 24.9% less than control rats at the end of the study. It appears that maitake lowers the risk of becoming obese to a certain extent.

The mushroom may be useful to people who want to lose weight or maintain their weight. In a study conducted at the Koseikai Clinic in Tokyo, 32 overweight subjects were given 10 grams daily of maitake powder for two months to see if they would lose weight. Without changing their diets, all subjects lost weight, with the average loss being 12 pounds.

One reason for weight loss may be that maitake curbs appetite, but losing weight often means losing stamina, energy, and strength. To obviate these problems and improve efficacy, a combination of effective appetite controllers with a mushroom known to deliver energy, *Cordyceps sinensis,* has been developed. The combination includes maitake, *Hoodia gordonii* (which helps the Bushmen of the Kalahari desert walk for days without craving for food), chromium polynicotinate (preserves the muscles), and *Cordyceps sinensis.*

Maitake and the Liver

The average person carries three to four pounds of bacteria in the gastrointestinal (GI) tract. Some of these bacteria are good for the body, helping to prevent constipation and diarrhea, for example. Bad bacteria, however, are also present in the GI tract. Certain types of bad bacteria produce a substance called D-galactosamine, which is associated with inflammation and liver toxicity. Physicians can determine how much damage has been done by D-galactosamine by testing for certain enzymes in the blood. If these enzymes are present in large amounts, the liver has been damaged.

In an experiment to see whether medicinal mushrooms can suppress the effects of D-galactosamine on the liver, scientists from Shizuoka University, in Japan, used D-galactosamine to damage the livers of laboratory rats. Then, they fed the rats various medicinal mushrooms for two weeks to find out which mushrooms might suppress D-galactosamine effects. Maitake worked best and the effects of maitake were dose-dependent. In other words, the larger the dose of maitake given to the rats, the better the effect it had on suppressing D-galactosamine.

This experiment seems to indicate that maitake can help protect the liver against the effects of bad nutrition. If you eat fast foods or foods that are low in fiber, taking maitake may be able to improve the health of your gastrointestinal tract and protect your liver from damage.

Maitake and the Immune System

Researchers have known for some time that 1-3 and 1-6 beta-glucans aid the immune system and that beta-glucans from different mushrooms aid the immune system in different ways. Maitake, for example, stimulates macrophages to produce more cytokines. Macrophages are powerful cells that engulf and destroy foreign organisms and substances, and cytokines are messengers that alert the immune system to the presence of an invader.

Scientists from the Tokyo University of Pharmacy and Life Science conducted *in vitro* experiments on a cytokine called tumor necrosis factor alpha (TNF-alpha). This toxin-like substance is especially adept at killing malignant tumor cells. What the scientists discovered is that macrophages release TNF-alpha only after they have eaten a certain kind of high-molecular-weight beta-glucan found in maitake. A study along the same lines conducted at Tokyo College of Pharmacy concluded that small-molecular-weight beta-glucan from the maitake mushroom serves to prime the cells of the immune system and get them ready for an attack. Yet another study from Tokyo College of Pharmacy looked at interleukin-6 (IL-6), another cytokine known for its effectiveness against tumor cells. This study noted that maitake stimulated the production of IL-6.

Researchers from Kobe Pharmaceutical University, the group led by Professor Nanba, demonstrated that the polysaccharide D-fraction of maitake activates macrophages, dendritic cells, and T cells, resulting in the inhibition of growth of tumor cells. They also found that D-fraction enhanced the cytotoxicity of natural killer (NK) cells through the production of interleukin-12 (IL-12) by the macrophages activated by the D-fraction. These results confirm the outstanding activity of the beta-glucans of *Grifola frondosa* on diverse compartments of our immune defenses, notably against cancer.

5

Shiitake

n the 1960s, Japanese researchers undertook a series of epidemiological studies to learn everything they could about incidences of disease in their country. In one study, they found two remote mountainous districts where cancer was nearly unheard of. The government sent teams of scientists to these districts to ascertain why cancer rates were so low there. Was it something about how the people lived? Something in the diet? It so happened that growing shiitake mushrooms was the chief industry in both districts, and the inhabitants ate a lot of shiitake, apparently believing that it helped prevent cancer.

The name *shiitake* comes from the Japanese word for a variety of chestnut tree, *shita*, and the word for mushroom, *take*. Shiitake is sometimes called the "Forest Mushroom" and the "Black Forest Mushroom." In China, it is known as *Shaingugu* (*pin yin = Shang Gu* or *Shiang-ku*), which means "fragrant mushroom"; also Hua Gu or Qua Gu, which means "white flower mushroom"; this is the name given to the cracked white "Donko" variety of shiitake. Shiitake's Latin name is *Lentinula edodes* (*lent* means "supple," *inus* means "resembling," and *edodes* means "edible"). About 1980, a debate concerning shiitake's Latin name broke out among taxonomists and the mushroom's name was changed from *Lentinus edodes* to *Lentinula edodes*.

After the white button mushroom, shiitake is the most popular culinary mushroom in the world. The cultivation of shiitake in the United States is increasing faster than the cultivation of any other culinary mushroom. The mushroom's meaty flavor can complement almost any dish and, as it turns out, the mushroom that delights so many with its distinctive flavor is also a medicinal mushroom. Even among mushrooms, shiitake is high in nutrition: it contains all the essential amino acids, as well as eritadenine, a unique amino acid that some physicians believe lowers choles-

Shiitake

After the white button mushroom, shiitake is the most popular culinary mushroom in the world. The mushroom's meaty flavor can complement almost any dish and, as it turns out, the mushroom that delights so many with its distinctive flavor is also a medicinal mushroom.

• Name: Latin name, *Lentinula edodes: lent* means "supple," *inus* means "resembling," and *edodes* means "edible." *Shiitake* comes from the Japanese word for a variety of chestnut tree, *shita,* and the word for mushroom, *take.* Sometimes called the "Forest Mushroom" and the "Black Forest Mushroom." In China, known as *Shaingugu* (or *Shiang-ku*), which means "fragrant mushroom." The name may derive from the *Shii* tree, Japanese for "oak"; the name shiitake would therefore mean "oak mushroom."

• Description: Cap is dark brown at first and grows lighter with age; spores are white and the edges of the gills are serrated.

• Habitat: Shiitake grows on dead or dying hardwood trees (chestnut, beech, oak, Japanese alder, mulberry, and others), during the winter and spring. Native to Japan, China, the Korean peninsula, and other areas of East Asia.

• Active ingredients: 1-3 beta-glucans; polysaccharide KS-2; glycoproteins (LEM, LAP); eritadenine; iron, niacin, vitamins B_1 and B_2.

• Uses: Major anti-cancer agent in Japan (Lentinan®); anti-viral (HBV, HIV); anti-bacterial (strep throat; fights caries); protects the liver; lowers cholesterol; helps control high blood pressure.

terol. Shiitake is also high in iron, niacin, and B vitamins, especially B1 and B2. In sun-dried form, it contains vitamin D. Hot water extracts from cultured mycelium of *Lentinula edodes* contain polysaccharide KS-2, a peptide containing the amino acids serine, threonine, alanine, and proline.

SHIITAKE IN THE WILD

The shiitake mushroom is native to Japan, China, the Korean peninsula, and other areas of East Asia. The cap is dark brown at first and grows lighter with age. The spores are white and the edges of the gills are serrated. In the wild, shiitake grows on dead or dying hardwood trees (chestnut, beech, oak, Japanese alder, mulberry, and others) during the winter and spring. It prefers forest shade where cold water is nearby. The shiitake industry in Japan, as large as it is, can be credited with preserving much of the nation's forests. Without income from shiitake, many a yeoman farmer would have long ago cut down his trees or sold his land to developers. Shiitake mushrooms are Japan's leading agricultural export. Japan used to account for 80% of worldwide shiitake production; China exports considerably more than Japan now. The city of Qingyuan is said to produce more than 50% of the world's shiitake crop.

CULTIVATING SHIITAKE

Shiitake cultivation in the United States got off to a slow start, thanks in part to the United States Department of Agriculture (USDA). For much of the last century, the USDA imposed a complete quarantine on the importation of shiitake mushrooms, because they mistook *Lentinus edodes* for another mushroom called *Lentinus lepideus*. This latter mushroom (its common name is "Train Wrecker") was known to attack and corrode railroad ties and was the suspect in several railway mishaps. The USDA realized its mistake and lifted the quarantine against shiitake in 1972. Today, American growers produce approximately 5 million pounds of shiitake mushrooms annually.

In nature, the shiitake fungus propagates and spreads from spores produced by the mushroom. However, for cultivation, spore germination is too unreliable. Instead, logs are inoculated with actively growing fungus. The fungus is first adapted to wood by growing it directly on small pieces of wood. Active fungal cultures intended as inoculum for mushroom cultivation are called spawn. Because the quality of the crop can be no better than the spawn, growers must use viable shiitake spawn of a good variety in pure culture, free of weed fungi and bacteria.

Immunomodulating activities of extracts from *Lentinula edodes* decrease rapidly when the mushrooms have been stored at 20°C for 7 days, while no decrease occurs at low temperature storage (between 1°C and 5°C). It is imperative that medicinal mushrooms be harvested when they contain the optimum beta-glucan concentration and that the harvested fruitbodies should be stored at the correct temperature before processing or consumption. Drying stops the beta-glucan loss.

THE LEGEND OF SHIITAKE

Historical documents in Japanese archives relate how Chuai, the bellicose 14th Emperor of Japan, praised the shiitake mushrooms that were given to him by members of the barbarian Kumaso tribe, whom he was trying to subdue on the island of Kyushu in the second century. Shiitake is supposed to have been used in the ancient Japanese royal court as an aphrodisiac.

In China, the cultivation of shiitake mushrooms began about 1,000 years ago with a woodcutter named Wu San-Kwung in the mountainous areas of Zhejiang Province. To test his axe, Kwung swung it against a fallen log on which shiitake mushrooms grew. Days later, he noticed shiitake mushrooms growing where his axe struck the log. As an experiment, he cut the log in several different places. Once again, shiitake mushrooms grew where his axe landed. In this way, the log method of cultivating mushrooms was born. On one occasion, the story goes, mushrooms failed to grow on a log and Kwung grew frustrated. He attacked the log, beating it vigorously with the blade of his axe. When he returned to the scene of the battering, he discovered to his surprise that the log was covered with mushrooms. Kwung had discovered the "soak and strike" method of mushroom cultivation, in which logs are battered in such a way that spores have more openings in which to germinate. This method is still used in some places. Wu San-Kwung's contributions to agriculture are commemorated in a temple in Qingyuan. Festivals in his name are still celebrated throughout Zhejiang Province.

RESEARCH STUDIES ON SHIITAKE

In traditional Chinese medicine, shiitake is used to treat high cholesterol, atherosclerosis, colds, and flu. The mushroom is also believed to enliven the blood, dispel hunger, and cure the common cold. It is supposed to boost *Qi*, the primal life-force that animates the body and connects it to the living cosmos, according to traditional Chinese medicine. Given the high regard with which shiitake is held, it was only a matter of time before scientists tested its medicinal properties.

Shiitake and Cancer

In 1969, Tetsuro Ikekawa of Purdue University, working in conjunction with researchers at the National Cancer Center Research Institute, in Tokyo, extracted a 1-3 beta-glucan from shiitake that he tested on mice infected with tumors. In 72% to 92% of the mice, tumor growth was inhibited. From this study, Lentinan® was born (the beta-glucan was named for *Lentinula edodes*). Ikekawa and his colleagues conjectured that Lentinan bolstered the immune system by activating macrophages, T lymphocytes, other immune system cells, and the production of cytokines.

By 1976, scientists had run clinical trials on Lentinan and produced a pharmaceutical version. The Japanese government's Health and Welfare Ministry, the equivalent of the United States Food and Drug Administration (FDA), soon approved the drug. Almost immediately, Lentinan proved effective in treating many kinds of cancer. However, the drug does not have any direct anticancer activity. When Lentinan is placed in a test tube with cancer cells, it does not affect the cells, but when it is injected into the body, Lentinan triggers the production of T cells and natural killer cells. Lentinan is the third most widely prescribed anticancer drug in the world. Doctors often prescribe it to patients who have undergone chemotherapy, as a means of revitalizing the patients' immune system. Regrettably, Lentinan has not been approved by the FDA; except under special circumstances, it is not available to Americans.

Lentinan is very safe: in antigenicity studies, there were no anaphylactic reactions and no allergic reactions. Lentinan had no effect in a mutagenicity test, hemolysis test, blood coagulation, or ability to induce arthritis.

Shiitake and Hepatitis

A substance extracted from shiitake called LEM (*Lentinula edodes* mycelium) is believed to be helpful against hepatitis B, a disease transmitted by blood transfusions, nonsterilized needles, and sexual contact. Some studies have shown that LEM stimulates the production of antibodies that counteract hepatitis. While Lentinan is a pure polysaccharide composed, LEM and LAP, also present in mycelial extracts of *Lentinula edodes*, are glycoproteins and have demonstrated antitumor activity in clinical trials. LEM and LAP extracts are derived from *Lentinula edodes* mushroom mycelium and culture media, respectively, and are glycoproteins containing glucose, galactose, xylose, arabinose, mannose, and fructose. LEM also contains nucleic acid derivatives, vitamin B compounds, and ergosterol. Again, both LEM and LAP activate the host immune system. In Japan, Lentinan is presently classified as a medicine, whereas LEM and LAP are considered as food supplements (nutraceuticals).

Shiitake and HIV/AIDS

Shortly after the AIDS epidemic began in the early 1980s, physicians began experimenting with Lentinan as a means of making the immune system less susceptible to HIV, the virus that causes AIDS. Lentinan generated a lot of enthusiasm at the Sixth International Conference on AIDS in 1990, when reports were published showing the drug's ability to increase helper T cells, the cells whose job it is to mark invaders so they can be destroyed by the immune system (HIV destroys helper T cells). Shiitake's lignins, found in LEM, have been shown to block HIV proliferation and protect T-helper lymphocytes. A novel protein designated lentin was recently isolated from *Lentinula edodes* by biochemists of the Chinese University of Hong Kong. It has potent antifungal activity, but it also exerted an inhibitory activity on HIV-1 reverse transcriptase, as well as on proliferation of leukemia cells.

Researchers in the United States were also curious whether Lentinan could be used to treat AIDS patients. The researchers wanted to know whether Lentinan could strengthen AIDS patients' immune systems and whether the patients would tolerate Lentinan as well as Japanese cancer patients had in earlier studies. The study of AIDS patients was conducted jointly in San Francisco and New York. At San Francisco General Hospital, 10 patients were intravenously administered 2 milligrams (mg), 5 mg, or 10 mg of Lentinan or a placebo, once a week for eight weeks. At the Community Research Initiative in New York, two groups of 20 patients were intravenously administered either 1 mg or 5 mg of Lentinan, twice a week for 12 weeks, and 10 patients were administered a placebo. In all patients who took Lentinan, the number of lymphocytes (white blood cells that help flush viruses and bacteria from the body) increased. However, researchers cautioned that the small number of patients in the study prohibited them from concluding that Lentinan actually increases activity by lymphocytes. Lentinan when used in conjunction with azidothymidine (AZT) suppressed the surface expression of HIV on T cells more than AZT did alone. Lentinan and sulphated lentinan exhibited a potent anti-HIV activity, resulting in inhibition of viral replication and cell fusion.

A subsequent trial in which the researchers treated some patients with Lentinan and didanosine and other patients with didanosine alone showed a marked increase in lymphocytes in the Lentinan-didanosine patients when compared with those who received only didanosine. These provocative studies suggest that Lentinan can be useful for treating patients with HIV.

Shiitake and Tooth Decay

Dental plaque is a soft, thin, sticky film that forms on the surface of teeth, often near the gum-line. It is made up of millions of bacteria, as well as saliva and other substances, and can cause tooth decay. In case you haven't heard by now, the best way to prevent plaque from forming on teeth is to brush regularly.

To see if shiitake can help prevent tooth decay, researchers from the Nihon University School of Dentistry, in Japan, conducted a test in which they exposed the *Streptococcus mutans* and *Streptococcus sobrinus* bacteria to shiitake powder. These bacteria are the primary components of dental plaque. In an *in vitro* test, researchers observed a decrease in plaque formation. In an *in vivo* test conducted on laboratory rats that had been infected with *Streptococcus mutans*, researchers compared rats who had been fed the shiitake extract with rats that did not get the benefit of shiitake. The researchers discovered significantly fewer cavities in the shiitake group. What's more, the shiitake component of the rats' diet amounted to only 0.25%, which indicates that shiitake may be a potent protection against tooth decay

In another study undertaken at the Nihon University School of Dentistry, researchers found that shiitake was effective against several bacteria, including varieties of *Streptococcus,* that are commonly found in the mouth. Generally speaking, the study found that microbes such as *Candida* that are not found in the mouth were resistant to the mushroom. It appears that as a medicinal mushroom, shiitake is especially useful to dentists.

Shiitake Protects the Liver

Both LEM and an ethanol extracted fraction of *Lentinula edodes* protected the liver of mice injured with dimethyl-nitrosamine. The liver enzymes were controlled and, more importantly, consequent fibrosis was prevented or averted. This antifibrotic activity in extracts from an edible mushroom should result in the development of protectors of the liver without side effects.

It has long been recognized that eritadenine, a compound extracted from *Lentinula edodes,* is able to lower blood serum cholesterol by accelerating the excretion of ingested cholesterol and its metabolic decomposition. Various studies have shown that *Lentinus* mushrooms can lower both blood pressure and free cholesterol in plasma.

Shiitake and Bacteria

An extract of *Lentinula edodes* demonstrated growth-enhancing effects on beneficial bacteria in the colon, *Lactobacillus brevis* and *Bifidobacteria breve*. The effective factor in the extract is considered to be the disaccharide sugar trehalose. The researchers suggest that the *Lentinula edodes* extracts can improve the beneficial intestinal flora of the gut and reduce the harmful effects of certain bacterial enzymes, such as beta-glucosidase, beta-glucuronidase, and tryptophanase, as well as reducing colon cancer formation.

The culture medium of *Lentinula edodes* mycelium was tested at the Institute for Biotechnology, in Szeged, Hungary, against a number of common bacteria and *Candida albicans*. The pure mycelium-free culture medium prevented reproduction and proliferation of *Streptococcus pyogenes, Staphylococcus aureus,* and other bacilli. The active substance was isolated and identified as lenthionine, an antibacterial and antifungal compound that is not toxic for human tissues. Oxalic acid is another agent responsible for the antimicrobial effect of *Lentinula edodes* against *Staphylococcus aureus* and other bacteria.

6

Reishi

The names by which reishi is known give an idea of how revered the mushroom is in China and Japan. To the ancient Chinese, the mushroom was called *lingzhi* (*ling qi* or *ling chi*), meaning "spirit plant." The Chinese character for *lingzhi* is composed of three logographic characters—one for "shaman," one for "praying for," and one for "rain." Reishi has been called the "Ten-thousand-year mushroom" and the "Mushroom of immortality" because it is said to promote longevity. Reishi, the name by which it is known in the West, comes from the Japanese. The mushroom is also called the "varnished conk" on account of its shiny appearance, and the "phantom mushroom" because it is so scarce in the wild.

The mushroom's Latin name is *Ganoderma lucidum: gan* means "shiny," *derm* means "skin," and *lucidum* means "brilliant." Reishi has been called the king of herbal medicines, with many herbalists ranking it above ginseng. The late Professor Hiroshi Hikino of the University of Tohoku, in Japan, a premier authority on Eastern medicinal plants, called reishi "one of the most important elixirs in the Orient."

In 1995, researchers isolated the DNA of *Ganoderma tsugae* and *Ganoderma lucidum* and found that it was hard to differentiate between the two species. An even more recent study found that *Ganoderma lucidum* from Asia was in its own group, whereas *Ganoderma lucidum* from Europe and the Americas was more closely related to *Ganoderma tsugae*. Further investigation into the molecular make up of these two species is needed. To make matters more complicated, there are two different types of reishi: one with the traditional wide, shelf-like fruiting body, and the other antler-shaped and known as Rokkadu-Reishi. The antler form of reishi was avidly sought after by ancient Taoists and appears prominently in artwork dating back centuries. These two types are rumored to have different healing charac-

Reishi

Reishi has been called the king of herbal medicines, with many herbalists ranking it above ginseng. Although some people use reishi to brew teas, the mushroom is usually taken for medicinal purposes only, as it has a very bitter, woody taste.

• Name: *Ganoderma lucidum* is from the Latin word *gan,* which means "shiny," *derm* means "skin," and *lucidum* means "brilliant." Also called the "Ten-thousand-year mushroom" and the "Mushroom of immortality."

• Description: Most distinguishing feature is its shiny lacquered look; has a kidney-shaped cap and sometimes the spores appear on the cap and give the appearance of sandpaper. The mushroom comes in six colors: red (*akashiba*), white (*shiroshiba*), black (*kuroshiba*), blue (*aoshiba*), yellow (*kishiba*), and purple (*murasakishiba*).

• Habitat: Found in dense, humid coastal provinces of China; favors the decaying stumps of chestnut, oak, and other broad-leaf trees.

• Active ingredients: Beta- and hetero-beta-glucans; ling zhi-8 protein; ganodermic acids (triterpenes)

• Uses: Analgesic; anti-allergic activity; expectorant and antitussive properties; bronchitis-preventative effect, inducing regeneration of bronchial epithelium; anti-inflammatory; antibacterial against *Staphylococci, Streptococci,* and *Streptococcus pneumoniae;* antioxidant; antitumor activity, enhanced natural killer cell (NK) activity, and increased production of interleukin-1 and interleukin-2; antiviral effect; enhances bone marrow nucleated cell proliferation; cardiotonic action, lowering serum cholesterol levels with no effect on triglycerides, enhancing myocardial metabolism, and lowering blood pressure; anti-HIV activity; general immunopotentiation.

teristics. All the *Ganoderma* varieties seem to have essentially the same pharmacologically active compounds and have been used in much the same way, including *Ganoderma oregonensis* and *Ganoderma applanatum.*

Reishi is not a culinary mushroom. Although some people use reishi to brew teas, the mushroom is usually taken for medicinal purposes only, as it has a very bitter, woody taste. Reishi is bitter because the mushroom contains 119 different triterpenoids, the aromatic substances that have anti-inflammatory, anti-tumor, and antiviral effects. However, the cultured mycelium of the mushroom is not bitter, so people who take it in powder or capsule form need not be bothered by a bitter flavor.

The ancient Chinese text *Shen Nong Ben Jing,* from about 500 CE, states that *Ganoderma lucidum* is "useful for enhancing vital energy, increasing thinking faculty and preventing forgetfulness." It can "refresh the body and mind, delay aging, and enable one to live long. It stabilizes ones mental condition." The importance of retaining memory into old age probably lies in the Taoist belief that sickness was caused by past transgressions and that the patient had to remember the transgressions, record them, and destroy the record. This belief placed a strong emphasis on memory in the maintenance of health and longevity.

Modern herbalists use reishi to treat a variety of ailments, including chronic fatigue syndrome and diabetes. It is believed to detoxify the liver and help cure hepatitis. Reishi can lower cholesterol, prevent the growth of tumors, and prevent blood clots. In traditional Chinese medicine, reishi is used to treat asthma, gastric ulcers, insomnia, arthritis, and bronchitis. The mushroom is supposed to be an antihistamine and has been known to ease the suffering associated with bronchial asthma and hay fever. A recent study conducted at Mount Sinai Hospital, in New York, concluded that a Chinese formula (ASHMI) in which *Ganoderma lucidum* was the prominent active factor, was as active as systemic corticosteroids to control asthma. The authors concluded that anti-asthma herbal medicine intervention appears to be a safe and effective alternative medicine for treating asthma. In contrast with prednisone, ASHMI had no adverse effect on adrenal function and had a beneficial effect on T lymphocyte balance, a major immunological benefit in asthmatic and allergic patients. Reishi is also used to alleviate the symptoms associated with stress.

Reishi is considered a tonic. As such, it can build energy and increase stamina, although many herbalists warn that it works as a sedative in the short term. It is believed that vitamin C assists the body in absorbing reishi. For that reason, many doctors and herbalists recommend taking vitamin C along with the mushroom.

REISHI IN THE WILD

In its natural habitat, the reishi mushroom is found in the dense, humid coastal provinces of China, where it favors the decaying stumps of chestnut, oak, and other broad-leaf trees. In Japan, it is usually found on old plum trees. The mushroom's most distinguishing feature is its shiny lacquered look. Reishi's lustrous, well-preserved appearance may have contributed to its reputation as an herb that promotes longevity. It has a kidney-shaped cap that does not rot or lose its shape after drying. Sometimes the spores appear on the cap and give the appearance of sandpaper. The mushroom comes in six colors: red (*akashiba*), white (*shiroshiba*), black (*kuroshiba*), blue (*aoshiba*), yellow (*kishiba*), and purple (*murasakishiba*). Mycologist Malcolm Clark speculates that these mushrooms will eventually be separated by taxonomists into different species because the morphology of the mushrooms is different. Red reishi is *Ganoderma lucidum,* the mushroom that is used for medicinal purposes.

The reishi mushroom is extremely rare and difficult to find in the wild. Because the husks of the spores are very hard, the spores can't germinate as readily as the spores of other mushrooms. To germinate, the right combination of oxygen and moisture conditions is needed. Fortunately, mycologists are now able to recreate favorable growth conditions. It can be cultured on logs that are buried in shady, moist areas. *Ganoderma lucidum* can also be inoculated onto hardwood stumps. Under commercial cultivation conditions, *Ganoderma lucidum* is normally grown on artificial sawdust logs. The mushroom that was once the provenance of the emperors of China can now be purchased in health food stores.

THE LEGEND OF REISHI

Reishi has a colorful past. According to legend, Taoist priests in the first century were the first to experiment with reishi. They are supposed to have included the mushroom in magic potions that granted longevity, eternal youth, and immortality. The Taoist priests of the period practiced alchemy and were known for casting spells and mixing concoctions. They were looked upon as magicians or wizards; by present-day standards, they might be considered charlatans. But, remember, alchemy was the beginning of chemistry, and shamans, who treated the sick by summoning the forces of nature to the aid of their patients, were the first doctors. A poem by the first-century philosopher Wang Chung remarks on the Taoist priests' use of mushrooms in their quest to attain a higher state of consciousness:

> *They dose themselves with the germ of gold and jade*
> *And eat the finest fruit of the purple polypore fungus*
> *By eating what is germinal, their bodies are lightened*
> *And they are capable of spiritual transcendence.*

Reishi achieved pride of place in China's oldest materia medica, the *Herbal Classic,* compiled about 200 CE. In characteristic Chinese fashion, the *Herbal Classic* divides the 365 ingredients it describes into three grades:

superior, average, and fair. In the superior grade, reishi is given first place, ahead of ginseng. To qualify for the superior grade, an ingredient must have potent medicinal qualities and also produce no ill effects or side effects when taken over a long period of time. The book says of reishi:

The taste is bitter, its atmospheric energy is neutral; it has no toxicity. It cures the accumulation of pathogenic factors in the chest. It is good for the *Qi* of the head, including mental activities. It tonifies the spleen, increases wisdom, improves memory so that you won't forget. Long-term consumption will lighten your body, you will never become old. It lengthens years. It has spiritual power, and it develops spirit so that you become a "spirit-being" like the immortals.

Reishi's reputation as the "Mushroom of immortality" reached Emperor Ti of the Chin Dynasty about 23 centuries ago. The Emperor is supposed to have outfitted a fleet of ships manned by 300 strong men and 300 beautiful women to sail to the East, where reishi was believed to be growing, and bring back the mushroom. The ships were lost at sea. Legend has it that the shipwrecked castaways washed ashore on an island and founded a new nation there. The island, the story goes, is called Japan.

In the *Pen T'sao Kang Mu* ("The Great Pharmacopoeia"), a 16th-century text, compiler Le Shih-chen had this to say about reishi: "It positively affects the life-energy, or *Qi* of the heart, repairing the chest area and benefiting those with a knotted and tight chest. Taken over a long period of time, agility of the body will not cease, and the years are lengthened to those of the Immortal Fairies."

In Chinese art, the reishi mushroom is a symbol of good health and long life. Depictions of reishi can be found on doors and door lintels, archways, and railings throughout the Emperor's residences in the Forbidden City and the Summer Palace. At various times in Chinese history, the Emperor's official scepter included a carving of a reishi mushroom. One Emperor's silk robe shows a peach tree, cloud forms, and, prominently, a reishi mushroom.

To the general population, the image of reishi appears to have been a good luck charm or talisman. In pen-and-ink drawings, tapestries, and paintings, subjects sometimes wear jewelry or jade pieces made in the image of the reishi mushroom. Kuan Yin, the Chinese goddess of healing and mercy, is sometimes depicted holding a reishi mushroom.

Some believe that the resurrection plant in the popular fairy tale "White Snake" is the reishi mushroom. In the tale, known to all Chinese children and the subject of operas and song, Lady White travels to faraway Kunlun

Mountain to obtain the resurrection plant and revive her deceased husband. By demonstrating her love for her husband, she wins the plant, and her husband lives again.

RESEARCH STUDIES ON REISHI

Reishi has been part of the Chinese pharmacopoeia for many centuries. Knowing its reputation as a healing herb, scientists began studying reishi in earnest beginning in the 1980s. Here are some of the most up-to-date studies on reishi.

Reishi and Skin Cancer

Aging doesn't damage the skin, sunlight does. Sunlight is not just light and warmth—it is also composed of ultraviolet light, which can penetrate the skin and cause all kinds of damage to blood cells, nerves, and even the eyes. Long periods of exposure to ultraviolet light can damage the skin's DNA. When the DNA is damaged and cannot recover, it may degenerate, and the result can be skin cancer.

To see if reishi can prevent this kind of damage and skin cancer as well, Korean scientists isolated DNA, placed it in an extract of the mushroom, and exposed it to ultraviolet radiation. They concluded that reishi shows "radioprotective ability" and guards against DNA damage. The experiment seems to indicate that eating reishi can slow the aging of the skin and protect as well against skin cancer.

Chinese women take reishi for beautification of the skin, and it is included in many Japanese patents for hair loss formulas, including products used for alopecia.

Reishi and the Side Effects of Radiation Therapy

Sometimes cancer patients are prescribed radiation therapy to kill cancer cells. However, radiation can have harmful side effects. Radiation damages DNA and has a hindering effect on the ability of blood cells to reproduce and proliferate. Radiation also kills blood cells, including the white blood cells that travel the bloodstream and fight infection. White blood cells are produced in the bone marrow. The part of the bone marrow that produces white blood cells is very sensitive to radiation. As a result, one consequence of radiation therapy is a reduction in the number of white blood cells that are produced. Having fewer white blood cells can be dangerous because it makes the body more susceptible to infection and disease.

To test whether reishi can aid cancer patients who have undergone radiation, scientists at Hebei Academy of Medical Sciences, in Shijiazhuang, China, did an experiment on laboratory mice. They irradiated the mice and then fed them spores from the reishi mushroom. The results of the experiment showed that reishi prevents the number of white blood cells from decreasing. Reishi also improved the survival rate of the irradiated mice. The experiment seems to indicate that reishi improves immune function by keeping the production of white blood cells from dropping in spite of radiation.

Reishi and Tumors

Essentially, the immune system can fight malignant cancer cells in three ways: cytotoxic T cells can kill the cancer cells outright; cancer cells can be weakened, allowing for the normal cells of the immune system to kill them; or substances similar to toxins can kill the cancer cells. Three of the toxin-like substances that have been associated with controlling the growth and survival of malignant cancer cells are as follows:

- Tumor necrosis factor alpha (TNF-alpha)

- Interleukin-1-beta (IL-1-beta)

- Interleukin-6 (IL-6) (Interleukins are messenger cells that allow the white blood cells to communicate with one another.)

To examine the immunomodulating and antitumor effects of reishi, scientists in Taiwan isolated polysaccharides from the fruit-bodies and tested them *in vitro*. The scientists discovered an increase in the production of the three toxin-like substances. The macrophages, monocytes, and T lymphocytes all increased their production of TNF-alpha, interleukin-1-beta, and interleukin-6. Interestingly, the increase in the three substances went to the upper level of the normal range. Too much TNF-alpha can kill normal cells, for example, but the reishi polysaccharides did not cause the production of TNF-alpha to rise to unsafe heights. This demonstrates the immunomodulating characteristic of reishi—the mushroom gives a push to the immune system, but doesn't overstimulate its activity.

Reishi also inhibits angiogenesis (development and growth of blood vessels that feed the cancer) in prostate cancer by modulating specific signaling. It is also one of eight herbs combined in a specialized formula known as PC-SPES, which has shown success in suppressing the symptoms of prostate cancer. It is also believed that reishi can induce the production of chemotherapy agents such as interferon (a protein that is produced inside cells to fight viral infection) and interleukin-1 and interleukin-2.

It inhibits growth, and induces actin polymerization, in bladder cancer cells *in vitro*. Furthermore, it inhibits the growth of breast cancer cells by modulating some signaling and could be an effective adjuvant in the treatment of this common cancer; this effect was found to be dose-dependent. An extract from mycelia of *Ganoderma lucidum* inhibited the growth of human hepatoma (liver cancer) cells, but not normal Chang human cell line. Six triterpenes have been sequenced at the Toyama Medical and Pharmaceutical University, in Japan.

Researchers in Taiwan have recently unraveled the mode of action of reishi polysaccharides. The research team was headed by Dr. Hsien-Yeh Hsu at the Institute of Biotechnology in Medicine, National Yang-Ming University, and Drs. Shui-Tien Chen, Chun-Hung Lin and Chi-Huey Wong at the Institute of Biological Chemistry and Genomics Research Center, Academia Sinica. The active component of reishi polysaccharides stimulates cytokine expression, and toll-like receptor 4 (TLR4) is one of the receptors. Various immune cells (including macrophages, B cells, dendritic cells, and stem cells) were also found to be activated by the active component of reishi polysaccharides. Natural killer (NK) cell–mediated cytotoxicity was also greatly enhanced and shown to effectively kill tumor cells when human umbilical cord blood cells were subjected to the treatment with these active polysaccharides.

Reishi as an Antioxidant

Recently, scientists at the Chinese University of Hong Kong isolated some substances in reishi that belong to the terpene group (some terpenes are anti-inflammatory). The scientists detected ganodermic acids A, B, C, and D, lucidenic acid B, and ganodermanontriol. These are all very powerful antioxidants, organic substances that counteract the damaging effects of free radicals on body tissues. Red blood cells carry oxygen and remove carbon dioxide, an essential process for the functioning of the body. However, if the red blood cells do not do their jobs correctly, oxygen can have damaging effects. Antioxidants help regulate oxygen use. From this excellent study, we can glimpse how reishi fortifies the body and helps the system stay in balance.

In 2004, a double-blind, placebo-controlled, cross-over study conducted at the Hong Kong Polytechnic University investigated the effects of 4 weeks of reishi supplementation on antioxidant status, coronary heart disease (CHD) risk, DNA damage, immune status, and inflammation, as well as markers of liver and renal toxicity. It was performed as a follow-up to a study that showed that antioxidant power in plasma increased after reishi ingestion, and that 10-day supplementation was associated with an improved CHD biomarker profile. In this study, fasting blood and urine from healthy adults (22–52 years old) was collected before and after the 4 weeks supplementation with a commercially available reishi preparation (1.44 g of reishi per day; equivalent to 13.2 g of fresh mushrooms per day) or a placebo. No significant change in any of the variables was found, although a slight trend toward lower lipids was seen and antioxidant capacity in urine increased. The results showed no evidence of liver, renal or DNA toxicity with reishi intake.

Anesthesiologists at Mackay Memorial Hospital, in Taipei, Taiwan, have recently demonstrated that an extract of *Ganoderma lucidum* had antioxidative effects against heart toxicity; it works as a superoxide scavenger of free radicals.

Reishi and Infections

A number of substances extracted from reishi have shown interesting anti-infective properties:

- A protein designated ganodermin is a potent anti-fungal agent.

- A proteoglycan is active against herpes simplex virus type 1 (HSV-1) and type 2 (HSV-2) by interfering with the early events of viral adsorption and entry into target cells. Ganodermadiol is active against HSV-1 causing lip blisters.

- Ganoderiol F and ganodermanontriol inhibited HIV-1-induced cytopathic effects at a very low concentration. Ganoderic acid B inhibits HIV-1 protease, while ganodermadiol possesses *in vitro* antiviral activity against influenza virus type A.

- Three new triterpenes inhibited Epstein-Barr virus, the cause of infectious mononucleosis and a tumor promoter.

Other Benefits of Reishi

Reishi is currently gaining the attention of Western medical practitioners because it has been shown to help treat coronary heart disease, hypertension, arthritis, and muscular dystrophy. (Combining the documented hypotensive effects of reishi, maitake, and *Cordyceps sinensis* may allow for an even more powerful synergistic healing effect, and could help a large number of patients at risk of stroke or heart attacks.)

Researchers found *Ganoderma lucidum* to be a potent anti-inflammatory agent in mice. The extract of the fruiting body was active orally against both carrageenan-induced inflammation, and croton oil–induced inflammation, two standard tests used on animals to study active anti-inflammatory medications. The extract was active as an anti-inflammatory agent both orally and topically. The active compound was equivalent in anti-inflammatory activity to hydrocortisone. However, it does not show the typical side effects of corticosteroids nor appear to cause stomach ulcers, a major side effect of nonsteroidal anti-inflammatory drugs, such as aspirin or ibuprofen.

Natural health practitioners in the West are beginning to use reishi for its sleep-promoting effects. Triterpenes in reishi are thought to be responsible for producing a calming effect on the nervous system. Also, the oil of the spores of reishi has prevented brain damage in a mouse model of Parkinson's disease. An extract of reishi inhibited the testosterone-induced growth of the ventral prostate in castrated rats, so it might well be a potential treatment for benign prostate hyperplasia (BHP), a common condition in aging men.

Reishi extracts have normalized blood pressure in a number of patients after four weeks. Reishi's oxygenated sterols inhibit the synthesis of LDL (or "bad") cholesterol better than statin drugs. Other triterpenes of the fungus contribute to atherosclerosis protection by inhibition of angiotensin-converting enzyme (ganoderic acid F) and of platelet aggregation (ganoderic acid S).

Beta-glucans (ganodelan A and B) help release insulin by facilitating the influx of calcium in the pancreas beta cells, lowering elevated blood sugar—a potential therapy for diabetes. Extracts of *Ganoderma lucidum* have shown good results in treating hepatitis, particularly in cases without severe liver impairment. A clinical study with an extract of *Ganoderma lucidum* showed highly beneficial results on quality of life in patients suffering from active hepatitis B.

Activation of the complement system, inducing the release of mediators from mast cells, can cause a variety of diseases and can be fatal if occurring after an organ transplantation. Several triterpenes from *Ganoderma lucidum* (ganoderiol F, ganodermanontriol, and ganodermanondiol) show strong anticomplement activity and are being tested in organ transplant patients. Other traditional benefits of reishi that have been confirmed by modern scientific research include inhibition of allergic reactions and relief from chronic bronchitis.

7

Cordyceps sinensis

n September 1993, a scandal broke out in the wake of the National Games in Beijing, China. In a single week, three women's track-and-field world records were broken. Never had a single track meet produced so many world records. Running the 10,000-meter race, Junxia Wang shattered the previous world record by an amazing 42 seconds (her record still stands). Two days later, the record in the 1,500-meter race was broken by Yunxia Qu, who completed the race a full three seconds faster than the previous record (Qu's record also stands). Then, in qualifying heats for the 3,000-meter race, giddy fans watched as the world record fell twice, first to Linli Zhang, who broke the record in the first heat, and then again to Junxia Wang, who broke her teammate's newly minted record in the second heat. On Friday, in the 3,000-meter final, Junxia Wang broke her own world record by six seconds (another record that still stands).

Some in the world of track-and-field cried foul. For so many world records to fall in one place in such a short time, the athletes must have been taking illegal performance-enhancing drugs. Surely when urine tests were completed, the results would show that the Chinese women had been taking anabolic steroids or some other illegal drug. But the urine tests were negative. If the athletes had taken drugs, the tests did not show it. When reporters pressed him on why his athletes ran so well, Coach Ma Junren mentioned their rigorous training schedule, their passionate commitment to track-and-field, and a secret elixir made from the *Cordyceps sinensis* mushroom.

The wonders of *Cordyceps sinensis* have been known in China for at least 1,000 years, where the mushroom is recognized as a national medicinal treasure, a precious and virtually sacred tonic. As a health supplement, it is known to increase energy and vitality. *Cordyceps* is one of the safest medic-

Cordyceps sinensis

The wonders of *Cordyceps sinensis* have been known in China for at least 1,000 years, where the mushroom is recognized as a national medicinal treasure, a precious and virtually sacred tonic. As a health supplement, it is known to increase energy and vitality.

• Name: The Latin etymology of *Cordyceps sinensis* is as follows: *cord* means "club," *ceps* means "head," and *sinensis* means "Chinese." The mushroom is also called the "caterpillar fungus" on account of its origin, and, less frequently, "winter worm, summer grass."

• Description: The mycelium is encased in the mummified body of the caterpillar, from which the fungus germinates. The fruit-body is capless, shaped like a blade or twig, dark brown at the base, and black at the top.

• Habitat: *Cordyceps* is found in the mountains of Tibet, as low as 14,000 feet and up to 21,000 feet high. Interviews with a number of local collectors suggest that none had ever seen it lower than the tree line, which is now around 14,000 in Tibet. It is usually found starting about 500 feet higher than the tree line. It may grow lower in Bhutan or Nepal, but in any case, it does grow above the 14,000 foot limit. It grows in the alpine meadows of the Himalayas and other high mountain ranges of China, Tibet, and Nepal.

• Active ingredients: Polysaccharides; deoxy-nucleosides (Cordycepin); other altered nucleosides such as hydroxy-ethyladenosine, which are antiviral and thought to work by a different mechanism than the deoxy-nucleosides.

• Uses: Anti-asthma and bronchitis; controls atherosclerosis (cardiovascular disease); lowers cholesterol; safely and effectively controls arrhythmias; helps control diabetes; antiviral (HIV, HBV); prevents liver cirrhosis (post-hepatitis); increases stamina and fights fatigue; increases libido and sperm count.

inal foods. The mushroom is used to treat liver diseases, cancer, angina pectoris, cardiac arrhythmias, bronchial problems, anemia, tuberculosis, jaundice, emphysema, infertility, and sexual dysfunction. In traditional Chinese medicine (TCM), *Cordyceps* is believed to nourish the *yin*, boost the *yang*, and invigorate the meridians of the lungs and kidneys.

The mushroom has a long and storied history in China. The first mention of *Cordyceps sinensis* appears in 620 CE during the Tang Dynasty. The literature describes a strange organism that lives high in the mountains of

Tibet and is able to change from animal to plant and back to animal again. That sounds far-fetched, but the ancient literature concerning *Cordyceps* is not as bizarre as it would seem. *Cordyceps sinensis* is indeed an unusual mushroom: it germinates in a living organism, the larvae of certain kinds of moths, chiefly the ghost moth or the bat moth (*Hepialus armoricanus;* the genus name was changed from *Hepialus* to *Thitarodes* some years ago, but both names are still used), which it mummifies, colonizes, and eventually kills.

The Latin etymology of *Cordyceps sinensis* is as follows: *cord* means "club," *ceps* means "head," and *sinensis* means "Chinese." The mushroom is also called the "caterpillar fungus" on account of its origin, and, less frequently, "winter worm, summer grass" because the ancient Chinese believed that the fungus was an animal in winter and a vegetable in summertime. Around 1850, Japanese herbalists began importing the mushroom from China and named it *tochukaso,* a Japanese translation of "winter worm, summer plant." The mushroom is sometimes called the "club-head fungus," a direct translation of its Latin name. The common name used in China today is *dong chongxia cao* (*chong cao* for short). In Tibet, it is called *yartsa gunbu,* which means "winter worm, summer grass."

CORDYCEPS SINENSIS IN THE WILD

There are over 680 documented varieties of *Cordyceps* mushroom, of which *Cordyceps sinensis* is but one. Many *Cordyceps* fungi grow by feeding on insect larvae and sometimes on mature insects. *Cordyceps* mushrooms grow on just about every category of insect—crickets, cockroaches, bees, centipedes, black beetles, and ants, to name a few. For example, *Cordyceps curculionum* attacks the body of ants and rides the ants high into the trees to disperse its spores.

In appearance, *Cordyceps sinensis* makes for an unusual sight. The mycelium is encased in the mummified body of the caterpillar, from which the fungus germinates. The fruit-body, sprouting from the caterpillar, is capless, shaped like a blade or twig, dark brown at the base, and black at the top. Large fruit-bodies sometimes seem to branch out in the manner of antlers (the reason why *Cordyceps* is sometimes called the "deer fungus"). The mushroom is now found at altitudes of 14,000 to 21,000 feet. It grows in the alpine meadows of the Himalayas and other high mountain ranges of China, Tibet, Bhutan, and Nepal.

Foraging for *Cordyceps*

In 1996, mycologist Malcolm Clark was privileged to accompany members of the Mykot tribe as they foraged for *Cordyceps sinensis* in the Himalayas. "The Mykots immigrated to Nepal long, long ago from Tibet," Clark explains. "Like all Nepalese, they keep yaks, but the yaks are herded, not fenced. At a certain time of the year, when the snowmelt comes, the yaks start heading up into the mountains and there is no way of holding them back. They climb up to 16,000 feet to find the *Cordyceps*. Most of the mushrooms we collected were collected between 12,000 and 14,000 feet." To prevent altitude sickness, Clark's companions urged him to eat the *Cordyceps* mushroom. "I ate fresh *Cordyceps* right out of the soil, because the Mykot told me it would help with altitude sickness. And I never got sick," Clark said.

"As the Mykot travel with the yaks, they look for a certain kind of primrose that blooms at high elevation. If the primrose isn't blooming, the *Cordyceps* is not going to be out, and you may as well turn around and go back because without the primrose there is no *Cordyceps*." Sure enough, when they came to where the primrose was growing, the yaks ate the grasses, the primrose flowers, and the *Cordyceps*, and the yaks began mating.

Recent *Cordyceps* Research Expedition to Tibet

In June 2006, Dr. John Holliday, director of research for Aloha Medicinals, a medicinal mushroom production company based in Hawaii and California, led one of the first formal, Western scientific research expeditions into the high country of Tibet in search of new strains of *Cordyceps*. They discovered what appear to be five previously unknown species of *Cordyceps*, closely related to *C. sinensis* and perhaps only subspecies or strains of this fungus. They appear different because they are growing on different species of caterpillars.

The remote villagers and nomads in the region knew of these different types and even have distinct names for them. Each type is ranked differently in terms of medicinal usage and value. There are *Cordyceps* that grow on white caterpillars, known as *Bu Carpo* in Tibetan, which are the lowest grade. Another *Cordyceps*, called *Go Marpu* in Tibetan, grows on a red-eyed caterpillar and is considered better than the *Bu Carpo* grade, but not as good as the top quality grade, known locally as *Yartsa Gunbu*. The price range

Among mycologists, there is a debate as to whether the *Cordyceps* fungus grows outside the caterpillar or is ingested and grows from the inside. Clark believes that the caterpillars actually ingest the *Cordyceps* spores. "When dissecting the caterpillars, I found color variation in the tissue always in more or less the same place. That leads me to believe that the spore is ingested. It gets down through the esophagus and into the gut of the caterpillar, where it germinates. You can actually see the spot of inoculation where germination takes place. I always find one spot on the larvae which is softer and a different color, so what I'm proposing is that it's ingested and it germinates from the inside, where it grows almost like a tuber. It splits the caterpillar's head and grows out through there. When the ground starts to warm in the spring, the *Cordyceps* breaks through the ground and the mushroom appears."

Clark's idea is that *Cordyceps* (the fungus itself) is actually composed of three different organisms. "The theory is that the three work together symbiotically. We may be talking about a yeast or another fungus. It has not been determined what these organisms are. I'm hoping there will be a breakthrough as far as separating the active parties."

---

between the different varieties is considerable. (There are also two other lower grades that are more uncommon and do not have their own Tibetan names.) Aloha Medicinals has managed to cultivate these different types in the laboratory and is currently investigating their various chemical and biological properties. Research will eventually determine the relationship between these different *Cordyceps* based upon the analysis of their DNA and other genetic parameters.

Dr. Holliday is also conducting research into *Cordyceps* from other areas of the world, particularly the high Andes mountains in Peru. There are about 250 newly found species of *Cordyceps* from Peru that have yet to be named by science. Some of these Peruvian *Cordyceps* have shown potent antibacterial and antiviral activities and are the subject of current research for the development of a new generation of nontoxic drugs for treating HIV and AIDS. Just how these species of *Cordyceps,* so remote from the classic Tibetan varieties, relate to one another is one of the questions for further research.

As more pharmaceutical companies expand into researching this medicinal mushroom, we will likely see many new drugs developed from this biologically active group of *Cordyceps* and other mushrooms.

The Mykots make a yogurt out of *Cordyceps*. They milk the yaks, skim the fat from the milk, and soak dried *Cordyceps* in the milk overnight. In the morning, the milk turns to yogurt. "Yogurt is typically made from *Lactobacillus* bacteria, which coagulates the proteins. But *Lactobacillus* is not present in the yogurt that the Mykot make from *Cordyceps*. Some kind of enzymatic action keeps it from happening. Perhaps *Cordyceps* yogurt presents an opportunity for a new health food product."

"Most of the collection spots we went to are hundreds of years old," Clark said about his expedition. "I accompanied the Mykots on the condition that I would not reveal where they harvest the *Cordyceps*. These were secret areas and I'm sure they wanted to blindfold me one or two times. It was a wonderful experience."

THE LEGEND OF *CORDYCEPS SINENSIS*

When spring arrives and the snow starts melting in the high mountains, the indigenous people of Tibet and Nepal, as they have done for centuries, take their yak herds to grazing lands at higher elevations. Arriving in the high country, the yaks feed on the fresh spring grass. They paw the ground and remaining snow to expose and eat the *Cordyceps* mushroom. Then, in a frenzy, they begin rutting. As the story goes, herdsmen who observed the yaks rutting in a fever pitch wondered what gave the animals their vitality. Did they eat some kind of animal aphrodisiac? The herdsmen wondered how the animals managed to conduct themselves so vigorously in spite of the high elevation, and they wondered if what was good for the yak might be good for them.

Upon close examination, the herdsmen discovered that the animals were eating an unusual mushroom, one that grew from the body of dead caterpillars. An intrepid tribesman decided to experiment for himself. He ate a *Cordyceps sinensis*, found the results satisfactory, and recommended it to his companions. Soon, all the tribespeople were eating the mushroom. Their stamina improved and they suffered less from respiratory and other illnesses. The tribespeople shared the newly discovered mushroom with monks of their acquaintance, who shared it with other monks, and soon the reputation of *Cordyceps sinensis* spread throughout China. Eventually, the miracle mushroom landed in the hands of the Emperor's physicians, who prescribed it for the Emperor. Thereafter, by decree, *Cordyceps* could be taken only in the Emperor's palace. All who obtained the mushroom were required by law to turn it over to officers of the Emperor.

Ancient texts describe a couple of unusual ways to take *Cordyceps*. One recipe called for the mushroom to be soaked in yellow wine to make a tonic for the relief of pain in the groin and knees. Another described preparing *Cordyceps* in the belly of a male duck. People suffering from cancer or fatigue were instructed to stuff 8.5 grams of a whole *Cordyceps* mushroom, with the caterpillar casing still attached, into the belly of a newly killed duck, and boil the duck over a slow fire. After the duck had been boiled, the patient was to remove the *Cordyceps* and eat the duck meat for 8 to 10 days until healthy. For more recipes see page 147.

CORDYCEPS: EAST AND WEST

For many centuries, *Cordyceps* has been the herb of choice in China for treating kidney and lung ailments. In traditional Chinese medicine (TCM), *Cordyceps* is said to go directly to the kidneys and lungs, the kidneys being the "root of life" and the lungs being the "*Qi* of the entire body." *Cordyceps* is considered a potent herb in the pharmacopoeia of TCM.

Lungs are thought to rule the *Qi*, which is associated with the element of air. *Qi* flows without obstruction through the lungs when the lungs are in a healthy state, but if the *Qi* current is impaired or obstructed by a throat or lung ailment, a defect in nothing less than the body's life force can result. What's more, because the throat is looked upon as door to the lungs and the home of the vocal cords, nose and throat disorders are treated by way of the lungs. For that reason, *Cordyceps,* which goes directly to the lungs and kidneys, is sometimes prescribed for nose and throat disorders.

The kidneys are judged as especially important in TCM because they store *Jing,* the prime organic material that is the source of regeneration in the body. All the organs of the body are completely dependent on the kidneys for their life activity. The natural weakening of *Jing* over time brings about old age. Erectile dysfunction, sterility, and reproductive problems are brought about when the kidneys do not store *Jing* properly. Kidneys control the bones and produce bone marrow, and even normal breathing requires the assistance of the kidneys. Because the kidneys are so central to Chinese notions of good health and bodily function, *Cordyceps,* the herb that goes to the kidneys, is prescribed for many ailments.

The West's first encounter with *Cordyceps* occurred in the early 18th century when Father Jean-Baptiste Perennin du Halde, a Jesuit priest, brought back specimens from China to his native France. During his stay in the Emperor's court, Father Perennin took a lively interest in *Cordyceps*.

Very likely, his curiosity about the mushroom came about when he was pre-scribed it during a grave illness. According to his diary, Father Perennin, very ill with a fever, had the good fortune to come upon an emissary to the Great Palace who happened to be delivering *Cordyceps*. The man offered Father Perennin the *Cordyceps* and he soon recovered.

In his diary, Father Perennin wrote that *Cordyceps* can "strengthen and renovate the powers of the system that have been reduced either by overex-ertion or long sickness." He noted how rare *Cordyceps* was in China, how it had to be imported from the mountainous kingdoms of Tibet, and how it was worth four times its weight in silver.

Upon his return to France, Father Perennin published an account of his experiences with *Cordyceps* and the beneficial effect it had on his health. His report caused a small sensation in the French scientific community. In his report, a mushroom had been shown to have an association with an insect for the first time. The discovery opened the door to the idea of using microorganisms to control crop pests.

The first indication of the origin of *Cordyceps* didn't occur in the West until 1843, when the Reverend Dr. M.I. Berkeley, writing in the *New York State Journal of Medicine*, solved the riddle of the mysterious insect-plant. Berkeley noted that the root of *Cordyceps* is indeed a caterpillar, but that the caterpil-lar had been taken over almost entirely by the mushroom's mycelium.

Cordyceps probably made its debut in the United States in the mid-1800s, when Chinese immigrants began arriving to build the railroads. Records show that Chinese physicians were prescribing *Cordyceps* in Ore-gon and Idaho. The first to market the mushroom were the Lloyd brothers of Cincinnati, Ohio, leading producers of herbal medicines in the United States at the turn of the 20th century. They solicited information about *Cordyceps* from a botanist in China named N. Gist Gee and used the infor-mation in their promotional literature. Gee explained that the mushroom was carried down from the mountains of Tibet by tribespeople who col-lected it at 12,000 to 15,000 feet. He wrote that Chinese doctors recognized it as "good for protecting the lungs, enriching the kidneys, stopping the flowing or spitting of blood, decomposing phlegm produced from persist-ent coughing, and curing consumption."

GETTING THE REAL THING

Beginning in the 1960s, Chinese mycologists undertook extensive research on *Cordyceps* with an eye toward isolating the most potent strain. Because

Cordyceps is rare and difficult to collect in the wild, their goal was to locate a superior strain to supply the ever-increasing worldwide demand for the mushroom. In 1972, researchers at the Institute of Materia Medica of the Chinese Academy of Medical Sciences developed, tested, and finally decided on a strain that they called *Cordyceps* Cs-4 (or simply Cs-4). The strain was chosen because it is closest to wild *Cordyceps* in the similarity of its chemical components and in its beneficial qualities as an herbal medicine. In fact, Cs-4 was simply more amenable to artificial cultivation than their Cs-1, Cs-2 or Cs-3 strains. While Cs-4 is thought by many people today to be superior due to the many papers written on Cs-4, in truth is that both the biotechnology processes and the strain isolation have come a long way in the last 30 years. There are many strains today with a closer chemical profile to the wild *Cordyceps* than Cs-4.

Gordyceps Cs-4 was isolated from natural *Cordyceps* found in the Qinghal Province, a remote area that was renowned for its *Cordyceps* for many centuries. Cs-4 meets rigorous standards for safety, grows rapidly using many different cultivation techniques, and resists contamination. More than 2,000 patients with various medical disorders were involved in clinical trials of Cs-4 in China. It became the first traditional Chinese medicine to be approved under China's new and stringent medical standards. In 1987, China's Ministry of Public Health approved Cs-4—or *Jinshuibao*, as it is known in China—for use by the general population.

With the opening of China to business with Western countries in the 1970s, many people in countries far from China were exposed to the benefits found in TCM. Along with this exposure came an increased demand for the herbal medicines used in that medical system. The great demand worldwide for *Cordyceps*, and the enormous cost of the wild collected variety, led to many unscrupulous manufacturers and distributors providing adulterated and counterfeit *Cordyceps*. Most of the Western world prefers their medicine to come in neat little capsules, rather than in the whole caterpillar form, which makes it easier for some suppliers to sell just about anything under the label of "Cordyceps." In an attempt to identify what "real" *Cordyceps* was, a group in California started analyzing all of the available *Cordyceps*, both commercial products and bulk raw material products, grown by nearly all of the cultivators and suppliers worldwide. What they found was disturbing: too many commercial samples imported from China were almost devoid of *Cordyceps*, while a number American products consisted mostly of the unconverted grain substrate upon which the *Cordyceps* is grown.

The methods for analyzing *Cordyceps* quality have not yet become standardized throughout the world. Every lab that is conducting this type of testing uses its own methods and standards. Almost all of the samples of wild *Cordyceps* have been shown to be very similar in chemical composition, but there is variation in the secondary metabolite compounds present in cultivated *Cordyceps sinensis* and other *Cordyceps* species. The nucleosides, and specifically the deoxy-nucleosides (e.g., Cordycepin), have been determined to be the most reliable indicators of potency, and many are found in no other organism, or at best, in a very limited number.

Most consumers of wild *Cordyceps* already know that it is normal practice for collectors to insert small segments of twigs or even pieces of wire into the body of the caterpillars to increase the weight. Many consumers of capsulated *Cordyceps* do not know what real *Cordyceps* even tastes or smells like. The Hong Kong Polytechnic University has analyzed some specimens of "*Cordyceps* Capsules" that contained nothing but rice flour, and other samples which contained nothing but nutmeg.

CULTIVATING *CORDYCEPS*

There are significant variations in quality from different strains and producers of *Cordyceps,* and one is left to wonder why. After all, a tomato is a tomato, no matter where it is grown. Yet, with *Cordyceps,* even the same strain (Cs-4) from different growers turns out to be different from a standpoint of active ingredients. It is first important to realize that there are two different methods used today in the cultivation of *Cordyceps.* In the method primarily used in China, known as liquid culture or fermentation, the organism is introduced into a tank of sterilized liquid medium, which provides the necessary nutritional components for rapid growth of the mycelium. The mycelium is then harvested by straining it out of the liquid broth and drying it, after which it can be used "as is" or further processed. Generally, in this method, the extra-cellular compounds exuded by the fungus during the growth cycle are discarded with the spent broth. This represents a major loss of bioactive compounds as many of the active ingredients are extra-cellular in nature and are found only in small concentrations in the mycelium.

The second cultivation method is the solid-substrate method, followed by most growers in Japan and America. The mycelium is grown in plastic bags or glass jars full of sterilized medium, which is almost always some type of cereal grain (usually rice, wheat, rye, or sorghum). After some period of growth, the mycelium is harvested along with the residual grain. While this is more easily mastered, one downside of this method is that the grain content could be greater than the mycelium content. Some of the grain by-products may in fact be beneficial or synergistic. A bonus to this method is that the extra-cellular compounds are harvested along with the substrate and mycelium.

Cordycepin is an example of one of the compounds that is primarily extra-cellular in nature. Many tests have been done on cultured *Cordyceps* mycelium for the presence of Cordycepin. In solid-substrate grown *Cordyceps,* there is usually Cordycepin present, while in liquid-cultured *Cordyceps* there is usually very little.

The substrate of choice for most Chinese growers is a liquid medium based upon silkworm residue, with added carbohydrates and minerals. This seems a logical choice, since this mushroom is found in nature growing on insects. Dried silkworm bodies are the by-product of an existing industry and have little other use. This silkworm-based substrate seems to yield a relatively high-quality product. The only problem is that in the United States, the FDA requires that mycelial products be produced on a normally consumed human food source. Silkworms do not fit into that category. They are also not available as a raw material source to most of the worlds *Cordyceps* cultivators.

The newest, most interesting *Cordyceps sinensis* culture substrate is antioxidant-rich organic purple corn that analytical tests have shown to increase the percentage of active compounds and increase growth rate. Purple corn (frequently referred to as "blue corn") is botanically the same species as regular table corn. By a twist of nature, this corn produces kernels with one of the deepest shades of purple found anywhere in the plant kingdom. Research has shown that purple corn contains cell-protecting antioxidants with the ability to inhibit tumors in rats. These antioxidant beneficial molecules are found in the final *Cordyceps* mycelium preparation grown on purple corn.

Using the above-described substrates, the complete chemical profile of the cultivated *Cordyceps* still will not approach that of the wild collected *Cordyceps* unless it is grown under very specific conditions. For the organism to produce the essential medicinal compounds, it needs to be growth-stressed through the absence of oxygen, a drop in temperature, and the total absence of light. Grain-grown mycelium will have anywhere from 5% to 20% fungal polysaccharides in the final product. (Manufacturers should put the levels of active components on the label. Or consumers should write to manufacturers for this information.)

RESEARCH STUDIES OF *CORDYCEPS*

Cordyceps has proven useful against a variety of diseases. The mushroom, which grows under trying conditions at high altitude, seems to impart some of its vitality and strength to the people who take it. The following are recent studies that have been done on the *Cordyceps sinensis* mushroom.

Cordyceps and Atherosclerosis

In predisposed individuals, a diet high in saturated fats can cause high cholesterol levels. Because most people have trouble managing their diets, it is difficult for these people to lower their cholesterol. Often, prescription drugs are needed, but patients can also take health supplements such as *Cordyceps* to bring down the level of cholesterol in their blood. *Cordyceps*, combined with rigorous exercise and a well-balanced diet, especially one rich in fish, can be a big help in managing atherosclerosis.

In general, *cholesterol* refers to the fatty, waxlike material that is produced by the liver to perform vital functions such as hormone production and cell renewal. The liver produces most of the cholesterol that the body needs, but some of it is also obtained from animal products. High-density lipoprotein (HDL) cholesterol is the so-called good cholesterol, which transports fats, or lipids, through the body so that they can't collect. So-called bad cholesterol, known as low-density lipoprotein (LDL) cholesterol tends to deposit fats on the blood vessel walls, where it can cause atherosclerosis. What's more, when LDL is deposited in the liver, it can cause fatty liver tissue.

Atherosclerosis is caused when fatty cholesterol deposits form on the artery walls. The artery walls scar and may grow thick with lesions and abrasions called fibrous plaques. The plaques may grow so large that they block the flow of blood to vital areas of the body. What's more, immune cells and muscle cells that normally serve to keep the arteries healthy find their way to the plaques instead. Cell debris also gets stuck in the plaques. Eventually, large clumps known as thrombi appear on the cell walls. When they break away and enter the bloodstream (embolism), a hole is left in the artery wall that can result in hemorrhaging and sudden death.

It appears that *Cordyceps* helps prevent atherosclerosis by decreasing the number of platelets that can get caught in the plaques. *Cordyceps* does this by reducing the viscosity of the blood. In one study, coronary heart disease patients were given 3 grams (g) of *Cordyceps* a day for three months. They showed a significant drop in blood viscosity and a 21% drop in total cholesterol.

Clinical studies have shown that *Cordyceps* can increase the amount of good (HDL) cholesterol and reduce the amount of bad (LDL) cholesterol. In the largest study conducted on *Cordyceps* and cholesterol, which took place in China, 273 patients received 1 g of *Cordyceps*, three times a day. Cholesterol levels dropped by 17% on average at completion of the eight-week trial.

Chinese physicians have also used *Cordyceps* to treat hyperlipidemia, a disease caused by high levels of fat in the blood. How *Cordyceps* acts to treat this disease is not well understood, but it does help people who suffer from high cholesterol. In two placebo-controlled trials conducted in China, patients 60 to 84 years old were given *Cordyceps* to see how the mushroom would affect age-related oxidation of fats in the bloodstream. After subjects took the *Cordyceps*, doctors discovered that their red blood cells had significantly higher levels of an enzyme called superoxide dismutase (SOD), one of the body's natural antioxidants. SOD rose to a level usually found in 17- to 20-year-olds.

The good news for people who suffer from high cholesterol is that researchers have discovered that lowering cholesterol levels restores the inner lining of the arteries and allows them to relax from the stiffened, plaque-infested state. Apart from administering cholesterol-lowering agents such as niacin and cholestipol, exercise can have a significant effect on cholesterol levels. In one study, 26 men with high cholesterol were asked to ride a stationary exercise bike three times a week. The men, all older than 46 years, rode the bike for different amounts of time according to their level of fitness. Twenty-four weeks into the exercise program, their cholesterol levels had dropped by 9%.

Cordyceps and Chronic Bronchitis

Chinese researchers have conducted numerous clinical trials of *Cordyceps* in the treatment of chronic bronchitis, In one study, patients between the ages of 55 and 60, who had been suffering from chronic bronchitis for about 12 years, were randomly divided into two groups. The 27 patients in the study group received 3 g of *Cordyceps* three times a day for four weeks. The control group received a similar amount of a berry extract called *Oleum Viticis negundo*, which is commonly used in China to treat coughs, colds, wheezing, and bronchitis. At the end of the study, 21 patients in the *Cordyceps* group found significant relief from their symptoms, whereas only eight patients in the control group felt any improvement.

A second one-month trial with 35 patients was completed the following year. Jiangxi Medical College reported that *Cordyceps* had helped as many as 90% of the patients, or 18 of the 20 people in the study group. This compared to a mere 20% improvement rate in the control group. Medical examinations showed a significant increase in lung function in the *Cordyceps* group, and patients experienced fewer bronchial spasms, cough spells, and incidences of airway resistance. There were also significant increases in maximum breathing capacity and forced expiratory volume tests, which measure the amount of air that a patient can expel in one second. The *Cordyceps* patients showed about 40% more capacity than patients in the control group.

A 1995 survey sparked a revival of interest in *Cordyceps* for the treatment of respiratory illnesses in China. Researchers at Jiang-Su Provincial Hospital reported preliminary findings in 100 respiratory disease patients, the majority of whom had chronic bronchitis complicated with pulmonary heart disease or emphysema. Following two weeks of treatment with *Cordyceps,* patients caught fewer colds, showed improved expectoration and cough, and had fewer asthmatic symptoms. In addition, patients reported relief from night sweats and their appetites began to return. Since the Jiang-Su survey showed that 92% of patients taking *Cordyceps* improved on one or more of these functions, it is logical to suppose that *Cordyceps* could help patients with other respiratory disorders.

Cordyceps and Asthma

Physicians in China commonly prescribe *Cordyceps* for the treatment of asthma. In at least one clinical study of *Cordyceps,* arranged by Beijing Medical University, *Cordyceps* proved to be beneficial for asthma. Fifty asthma patients, 17 to 65 years old, had all had been unsuccessfully treated with antibiotics and other commonly prescribed Western medications. Thirty-two patients assigned to the *Cordyceps* group received 3 g of *Cordyceps* or 10 milligrams (mg) of the antihistamine astemizole for 10 days. Researchers reported that the total effective rate for the *Cordyceps* group was 81.3%: forced expiratory volume test scores improved in 10 patients, and another 16 patients had increased their scores by 20%. Subjects in the antihistamine group showed a total effective rate of 61.3% and treatment was not at all effective in seven patients. For patients in the *Cordyceps* group, it took an average of only five days to improve; but it took nine days for cough to subside in the antihistamine group.

Cordyceps and Cardiac Arrhythmias

Cardiac arrhythmia is a disturbed or abnormal heartbeat. The most common type of arrhythmia, atrial fibrillation, affects more than 2 million Americans; 15% to 20% of strokes in the United States are caused by atrial fibrillation. The disease has many causes, including acute intoxication, hyperthyroidism, and rheumatic valvular disease. Medications such as antipsychotic drugs and antidepressants can increase the risk of arrhythmias, as can high doses of nicotine, caffeine, and other stimulants. Some studies show that blood anticoagulants such as aspirin and warfarin may prevent stroke in arrhythmia patients.

In 1994, a clinical trial was undertaken at Guangzhou Medical College, in China, to see whether *Cordyceps* could be used to treat ventricular arrhythmia. The 64 subjects were assigned at random to two groups: the test group was given 1,500 mg of *Cordyceps* every day for two weeks, and the other group received a placebo. More than 80% of patients who were given *Cordyceps* improved, whereas only 10% of patients in the placebo group recovered. The remaining patients showed no change.

In another study at Guangzhou Medical College, patients with arrhythmia took 1,500 mg of *Cordyceps* per day for two weeks. An amazing 78% of subjects showed improvement. Doctors undertook another trial on 38 elderly patients to see how *Cordyceps* would affect them. This time, subjects took 3,000 mg of *Cordyceps* per day for three months. Of 24 patients suffering from supraventricular arrhythmia, 20 showed improvement, with their electrocardiograms (EKGs) demonstrating a partial or complete recovery. The medical status of three patients who suffered from a complete blockage of the right branch of the cardiac nervous system also improved. From this study, researchers concluded that the benefits of *Cordyceps* increase over time: the longer a patient takes it, the more his or her condition will improve.

Researchers at the Department of Internal Medicine at Hunan Medical University, in China, undertook a clinical study in 1990 on 37 arrhythmia patients to see if wild *Cordyceps* could help them. Nineteen patients were cured, six in the first week and 13 in two to three weeks, while the remaining 11 patients showed no improvement.

Cordyceps and Diabetes

Diabetes, an autoimmune disorder, is associated with abnormally high blood sugar levels. Autoimmune disorders occur when the immune system fails to distinguish between what does and what doesn't belong in the body. In the case of diabetes, T cells incorrectly attack the cells of the pancreas that produce the sugar-regulating hormone insulin, with the result that the body cannot control the buildup of blood sugar. *Cordyceps,* by calming and quieting the cells of the immune system, may be able to help against autoimmune disorders such as diabetes. However, research into the treatment of diabetes with *Cordyceps* has just begun.

The first experiments in treating diabetes with *Cordyceps* were undertaken in Japan and China in the 1990s, when scientists reported significant hypoglycemic, or sugar-lowering, effects from the mushroom. In one clinical study involving 42 diabetics, 20 received an herbal formula that included mycelium powder from *Cordyceps,* and the remaining 22 received the herbal formula only (the researchers did not say what ingredients were in the formula). After 30 days, in the *Cordyceps* and formula group, improvement was seen in 95% of cases (only one diabetic did not improve). Researchers ran tests for proteinuria (urinary excretion of proteins), which is a general indicator of disease advancement. Its presence in diabetics can mean the development of secondary complications such as kidney disease, liver disease, and heart disease. Researchers found a 16.7% increase in the rate of proteinuria in the formula-only group, while only half the diabetics in the *Cordyceps* group showed any evidence of proteinuria.

Cordyceps Cs-4 is effective in lowering both blood glucose and plasma insulin, improving glucose metabolism by enhancing insulin sensitivity, and improving oral glucose tolerance. It appears to lower blood sugar levels through specific polysaccharides (CS-F10 and CS-F30). However, patients who tend to be hypoglycemic should use the mushroom only after careful consultation with a physician. If you have a tendency to fatigue or anorexia, your blood sugar levels may already be too low. Taking *Cordyceps* may intensify this problem and cause unwanted health complications.

Recent research has focused on the synergistic effects of combining *Cordyceps sinensis* with other mushroom extracts, such as maitake and *Coprinus comatus.* Other hypoglycemic agents, such as the herb *Salacia oblonga,* biotin, chromium polynicotinate, and cinnamon, may also be added. These components have demonstrated activity in controlling high blood sugar, as well as anti-diabetic properties. This approach may prove beneficial for those with hyperglycemia.

Cordyceps and Hepatitis B

Hepatitis B is usually contracted by infected blood or sexual contact. It is the number one cause of liver cancer, chronic hepatitis, and cirrhosis of the liver. A vaccine for hepatitis B is available, but it is too costly for most people who live in Africa, Southeast Asia, and China, where the disease is most prevalent. In those parts of the world, an estimated 8% of the population will die from hepatitis B, and over 50% of the population will contract the disease in their lifetime. About 350 million people worldwide are believed to suffer from hepatitis B, according to the World Health Organization. An estimated 1 million people die each year from the disease. In the United States, approximately 1.25 million people suffer from chronic hepatitis B.

Even when the immune system is able to destroy infected cells and stop the hepatitis B virus from replicating, certain immune cells called cytotoxic T lymphocytes may act against the virus without destroying infected cells in the liver. In this case, something more is needed to prevent infected cells from becoming cancerous, especially in chronically infected people. The immunostimulant alpha-interferon is the main treatment for hepatitis B, but it is costly and effective in only about 30% of cases.

There is evidence that *Cordyceps* can treat some cases of hepatitis B. In one study, 83 subjects, 2 to 15 years old, who carried the hepatitis B virus but showed no symptoms were given *Cordyceps* for three months. A complete conversion of antibodies to the virus was found in 33 of the test subjects, which indicates that the infection had been completely resolved and the virus was no longer contagious. Meanwhile, researchers reported that the number of antibodies positive for the virus had decreased in 47% of the subjects. Because the subjects were so young and their immune systems were not as developed, the drop in the number of positive antibodies indicates that the benefits of *Cordyceps* may have been more significant than the study showed. Researchers believe that the greater a person's immune response, the less likely he or she is to become a chronic carrier of hepatitis B. Only 3% to 5% of the adults exposed to hepatitis B become chronic carriers, because their immune systems are developed, whereas 95% of infected newborns become chronic carriers. In children under the age of 6 years, about 30% become chronic carriers. The drop of 47% indicated by the study is indeed significant.

In 1990, a study was undertaken in which 32 hepatitis B sufferers were given 3,750 mg of *Cordyceps* a day for 30 days. Positive antibodies to the virus changed to negative in 21 patients. In 23 patients, tests showed that liver function had improved.

Cordyceps and Cirrhosis

Cirrhosis of the liver is a degenerative disease that is caused by scar tissue in the liver. People who drink alcohol to excess or suffer from hepatitis are subject to the disease. Sufferers are 100 times more likely to develop liver cancer. About 30% of sufferers eventually succumb to liver cancer or complications as a result of chronic active hepatitis B.

Cordyceps has proved to be beneficial to patients suffering from post-hepatitis cirrhosis, which sometimes results when the liver does not heal correctly after a bout of hepatitis. In 1986, an extract of cultured mycelium was tested in 22 patients with post-hepatitis cirrhosis. Patients took 6–9 g of *Cordyceps* every day for three months, and by the end of the study their symptoms had improved dramatically. Cirrhotic cells had disappeared in 15 patients and had decreased significantly in another 6 patients.

In a more recent study, Japanese and Chinese researchers found that mice developed a high-energy state in their livers, without signs of toxicity, after consuming large quantities of *Cordyceps* mycelium. The researchers concluded that one of the main effects of taking *Cordyceps* on a repeated basis might be a higher metabolic state of the liver. One drug prescribed to treat cirrhosis, called malotilate, helps the liver regenerate by activating the cells of its energy factories. This in turn boosts concentrations of adenosine triphosphate (ATP), which supplies energy to cells. The fact that *Cordyceps* increases ATP levels may be one way it helps repair the liver.

Cordyceps and Kidney Failure

Cordyceps can relieve acute kidney failure brought on by an adverse toxic reaction to antibiotics. Studies have shown that *Cordyceps* has significant kidney-protective effects against gentamycin and another aminoglycoside known as kanamycin. In a controlled study of patients who had developed a condition called gentamycin kidney toxicity, half the patients were given an extract of the cultured mycelium of *Cordyceps* while still taking gentamycin. The control group continued to receive the gentamycin and additional drugs to neutralize its toxicity. By the sixth day, 89% of the *Cordyceps* group had made a complete clinical recovery from the toxicity of gentamycin; in comparison, only 45% of the control group recovered.

In 1995, researchers in China reported that *Cordyceps* can help patients with chronic renal failure (CRF). A clinical study of 37 CRF patients treated with 5 g daily of *Cordyceps* for 30 days found significant improvement. Compared with the results of pre-treatment tests, red blood cell and hemoglobin counts were greatly increased. The most improvement was shown in the creatinine clearance test, which measures the kidney filtration rate in terms of waste product called serum creatinine. Tests showed an improvement rate of about 39%. In addition, there was a 34% decrease in blood urea nitrogen (BUN); a high level of BUN is a major indicator of kidney disease. The test subjects also showed increased levels of superoxide dismutase (SOD), one of the body's strongest free-radical scavengers. Equally important was the 63% drop in proteins found in the urine, which is one of the strongest indicators of an overall correction of kidney function.

Cordyceps and Kidney Transplants

Cordyceps provides protection against the toxicity of cyclosporine, the major drug used to prevent the immune system from rejecting newly transplanted organs. Cyclosporine is a very useful immunosuppressant that has transformed the field of transplantation and saved many lives. But because of its deleterious effect on the kidneys, the drug presents a difficult problem for transplant patients who rely on it for survival. By constricting blood vessels and causing damage to kidney cells, cyclosporine can induce acute kidney failure. It can also cause diabetes, hypertension, and malignancies, and make patients susceptible to infections.

In one clinical study on *Cordyceps,* researchers selected seven kidney-transplant patients who were taking the conventional cocktail of anti-rejection drugs—azathioprine, cyclosporine, and prednisone. All the subjects had developed low levels of infection-fighting white blood cells and other symptoms of organ rejection. *Cordyceps* was administered as a replacement for the toxic azathioprine. Researchers determined that *Cordyceps* had caused no inhibition of the leukocytes. In fact, their levels returned to normal, allowing the immune system to combat infections.

A larger, placebo-controlled clinical study of *Cordyceps* in kidney-transplant patients was conducted at Nanfang Hospital and Taizhou Medical School, in China, to test its ability to protect the kidneys from cyclosporine toxicity. Sixty-nine stable kidney-transplant patients were randomly assigned to two groups: one group of 39 patients received a placebo, while the other 30 patients received *Cordyceps*. All the patients received cyclosporine, and thoughout the 15-day trial, they were monitored for signs of kidney toxicity. Researchers found less kidney toxicity in the *Cordyceps* group, and the longer patients took the mushroom powder, the less toxicity there was. Based on their findings, the doctors who conducted the trial now recommend *Cordyceps* for kidney-transplant patients on cyclosporine. It is interesting to note, that cyclosporine is produced by another species of *Cordyceps, C. subsessilus,* or at least its anamorphs.

Cordyceps and Fatigue

Chinese athletes have begun to use *Cordyceps* as general health supplement to increase vitality and energy and as a post-exercise recovery food. In TCM, doctors have long used the mushroom to treat cases of excessive tiredness. *Cordyceps* seems to increase patients' stamina. For this reason, physicians have recently been looking into whether *Cordyceps* can aid patients who suffer from chronic fatigue syndrome.

Although the disease is a recognized disorder, chronic fatigue syndrome is difficult to diagnose accurately. Its strong psychological component has made it a controversial subject in Western medicine. No single test or biological aspect has yet determined the presence of chronic fatigue syndrome, and the biochemical and biological signs of the disease continue to be a subject of debate. Complicating the problem of diagnosis, fatigue can be caused by any number of diseases, including low blood pressure, AIDS, tuberculosis, depression, or hepatitis.

By definition, a person is diagnosed with chronic fatigue syndrome if he or she exhibits these symptoms:

• Shows signs of the disease for more than six months.

• Is not tired by reason of overexertion.

• Can get no relief by resting.

• Suffers from at least four of the following ailments: headache, muscle pain, unrefreshing sleep, memory impairment, inability to concentrate, post-exertion malaise, sore throat, multijoint pain, or tenderness of the axillary lymph nodes or cervical nodes.

More research needs to be done to determine the effectiveness of *Cordyceps* in alleviating fatigue. In the meantime, people suffering from fatigue who have tried *Cordyceps* have reported some encouraging results. How does *Cordyceps* help people who suffer from chronic fatigue? Scientists report that chronic fatigue sufferers have an unusual form of adrenal insufficiency and, strangely, high levels of male hormones. Because *Cordyceps* improves the function of the adrenal cortex, it may help people who suffer from chronic fatigue. The mushroom also strengthens the resiliency and integrity of the HPA (hypothalamic-pituitary-adrenal) axis, the neuroendocrine system that responds to stressful events by producing chemical messengers that bring feelings of despair. It appears that *Cordyceps* calms the HPA axis and thus the nervous system.

In any case, *Cordyceps* does appear to boost the stamina of people who are not suffering from chronic fatigue. At the annual meeting of the American College of Sports Medicine in 1999, Christopher Cooper, professor of medicine and physiology at the University of California—Los Angeles School of Medicine, presented a study that showed *Cordyceps sinensis* increases exercise performance. In the study, 30 healthy elderly patients underwent a double-blind, placebo-controlled trial in which they were tested on a stationary bike. Subjects who took *Cordyceps* increased their oxygen intake from 1.88 to 2.00 liters per minute; those who took the placebo showed no increase in oxygen intake. Dr. Cooper concluded, "These findings support the belief held in China that *Cordyceps sinensis* has potential for improving exercise capacity and resistance to fatigue. The results complement other studies which have shown increased cellular energy levels through the use of *Cordyceps*."

Recent studies addressed the underlying mechanisms by which *Cordyceps* improves or increases performance. It increases the ratio of adenosine triphosphate (ATP) to inorganic phosphate in the liver by a 45% to 55%. One double-blind study, published in the *American Journal of Clinical Nutrition* in 2000, tested the energy and endurance in 110 healthy, but sedentary adults. Half took 3 g of *Cordyceps* daily, while the other half took a placebo. After 12 weeks, the *Cordyceps* group could cycle 2.8% longer than they could before taking the supplement, while the placebo group decreased the length of their rides by 5.6%.

Cordyceps and Erectile Dysfunction

Cordyceps, which acts on the libido over a period of weeks or months, can be classified as a sexual restorative. Its use as a remedy for sexual dysfunction has a long history in China: *Cordyceps* was simmered with other herbal

medicines or cooked with meats such as lean pork, chicken, or steamed turtle, each of which was thought to have its own power to enhance sexual
function.

Using Western scientific methods, researchers have determined that
Cordyceps stimulates activities in the body similar to those produced by the
natural sex hormones. In 1995, laboratory research in Japan demonstrated
that *Cordyceps* mycelium extract inhibits muscle contractions of the double
chamber inside the penis called the *corpus cavernosum*, which consists of
arteries, veins, and muscle tissue. Under a relaxed, sexually stimulated
state, blood pours into this sponge-like structure and becomes trapped,
resulting in an erection.

Western-trained physicians in China have performed multiple studies
with *Cordyceps* in the treatment of male impotence. At Hua Shan Hospital,
in Shanghai, researchers tested the mycelium product in 286 impotent men.
After taking 1 g of *Cordyceps* three times a day for 40 days, 183 patients
reported improvement in sexual functioning. At the end of another 40 days,
almost half the men reported that their sex lives had been partially or completely restored.

When word got out, others wanted to begin their own trials. The Shanghai Institute of Endocrinology tried two 20-day courses of *Cordyceps* in 50
impotent men. After they had completed both courses of the mycelium, 13
patients reported that they had been able to resume sexual activity; another 12 subjects indicated that they were experiencing sexual sensations and
were now able to have erections.

8

Agaricus blazei

One of the most exciting medicinal mushrooms is a relative newcomer, *Agaricus blazei*. Many scientists believe that the beta-glucans in this mushroom are more potent than that of other mushrooms. The main beta-glucan in *Agaricus blazei* is the 1-6 form, with a spiral closely replicating the size and form of normal DNA. Forty years ago, the medicinal properties of the mushroom were known only to a few thousand villagers in Brazil, but since the world discovered the mushroom, its reputation has spread far and wide. *Agaricus blazei* has shown real promise as an immunomodulator and a defense against tumors.

Agaricus blazei does not have as colorful a past as some of the other mushrooms described in this book. Instead of the exotic East, the origins of *Agaricus blazei* can be traced to a small mountain town in Brazil called Piedade, located 120 miles (200 km) southeast of São Paulo. For centuries, the inhabitants of the town and its environs have savored a mushroom that they call *Cogumelo de Deus* ("the mushroom of God"), *Cogumelo do Sol* ("the sun mushroom"), *Cogumelo Princesa* ("the princess mushroom"), or *Cogumelo da Vida* ("the mushroom of Life").

In the summer of 1965, a Brazilian farmer of Japanese descent named Takahisa Furumoto was roaming the mountains outside Piedade when he found an unfamiliar but tasty mushroom. The mushroom appeared to be of the *Agaricus* family. Furumoto sent spores of the mushroom to Inosuke Iwade of the Iwade Research Institute of Mycology, in Japan. To learn more about the mushroom, Iwade, a scholar in the field of mushroom cultivation, attempted to grow the mushroom in his laboratory, an attempt that would take nearly a decade.

Meanwhile, back in Piedade, a group of scientists led by Dr. W.J. Cinden of Pennsylvania State University had begun their own investigation

Agaricus blazei

Many scientists believe that the active ingredients in *Agaricus blazei* are more potent than that of any other mushrooms. It has shown real promise as an immunomodulator and a defense against tumors.

• Name: Also known as Murrill's agaricus, Royal sun agaricus, and, less frequently, gee song rong and almond-flavored portobello.

• Description: Range in color from off-white to light brown; the caps emerge as round "buttons" from the soil and grow in size from one to 12 inches across, depending on the strain. At first, the gills are off-white, but within days they turn pink, purple, and then black.

• Habitat: Originally from a small mountain town in Brazil called Piedade, located 120 miles southeast of São Paulo; grows in the southeastern United States, although not as prolifically as in South America. It is closely related to the North American *Agaricus subrufescens,* which may turn out to be the same species; this in turn may be good news, since this species is cultivated and available fresh at some local markets in the U.S.

• Active ingredients: Beta-(1-3)-D-glucan; beta-(1-4)-a-D-glucan; beta-(1-6)-D-glucan; RNA-protein complex; glucomannan.

• Uses: Increases production of interferon and interleukins; fights cancer metastases (uterus); reduces high blood pressure, blood glucose, cholesterol levels, and the effects of arteriosclerosis; anti-inflammatory and anti-allergic.

into the unknown *Agaricus* mushroom. Dr. Cinden and his colleagues had come to Piedade to find out why the inhabitants of the town had low rates of geriatric diseases and a reputation for longevity. He concluded that the people of Piedade enjoy long life because they eat an unusual mushroom of the *Agaricus* family as part of their diet. He published his findings in *Science* magazine and presented his conclusions at several conferences. Word about the unusual mushroom from Brazil began to spread.

After Inosuke Iwade at last managed to cultivate samples of the *Agaricus* mushroom in his laboratory in Japan, he noticed that this *Agaricus* was longer and thicker than others in the *Agaricus* family. The gills took longer than usual to turn black, the mushroom emitted a strong aromatic odor, and the root was sweet and delicious. Did he have a new species on his hands?

Iwade submitted a sample of the mushroom to a Belgian taxonomist named Heinemann, who deemed the mushroom a new species of *Agaricus*. He named it *Agaricus blazei* Murrill because, as it turned out, the mushroom had already been documented and described by the noted American mycologist W.A. Murrill.

The story is probably a fabrication to render the healing powers of this mushroom more plausible. In reality, the inhabitants of Piedade have never eaten this mushroom, which is, today, not even common in their area. Furumoto was rather captivated by its excellent organoleptic properties, which reminded him of the famous matsutake, a delicious edible but rare mushroom in Japan. He therefore sent samples of the Brazilian mushroom to several Japanese universities, and he also consulted the well-known Belgian agaricologist, Paul Heinemann, who identified the species as *Agaricus blazei* Murrill. Subsequently, after 10 years of sustained efforts, Japanese mycologists managed to cultivate the mushroom. A literature search reveals that the medicinal properties of this mushroom have mainly been studied by Japanese pharmacologists. Not surprisingly, it is also Japanese companies who have marketed *A. blazei*–based medicinal drugs.

William A. Murrill had found the mushroom in 1945 on the lawn of his friend R.W. Blaze, who lived in Gainesville, Florida. For years, this new mushroom, which is unknown in Europe and far from common in North America, remained in the dark until it was rediscovered in the 1960s by Japanese coffee growers working in Brazil. From the 1930s until his death in 1957, Murrill discovered over 650 species of fungi.

AGARICUS BLAZEI IN THE WILD

Agaricus mushrooms are quite common throughout the world—there are about 30 species. The "button mushroom" (*Agaricus bisporus*) found in American supermarkets is an example of an *Agaricus* mushroom. The mushrooms range in color from off-white to light brown. The caps emerge as round "buttons" from the soil and grow in size from one to 12 inches across, depending on the species. At first the gills are off-white, but within days they turn pink, purple, and then black. Chances are, if you see a mushroom growing on a lawn or in a pasture, it is an *Agaricus* mushroom.

Agaricus blazei, however, does not grow as wantonly as most *Agaricus* mushrooms. Where other species of mushroom prefer shade and dampness, *Agaricus blazei* favors the humid, hot-house environment of its native Brazil. The mushroom grows only in the hot summer months, and it may die if temperatures drop too low. In the Piedade region, temperatures range from 95 °F (35 °C) during the day to 72 °F (22.2 °C) at night, and the land receives a good dousing by tropical rain in the afternoon or early evening. According to a story, one reason that *Agaricus blazei* thrives in the region has to do with the number of wild horses found there. Horse manure, the story goes, contributes to the fertility and unique composition of the soil.

Agaricus blazei grows in the southeastern United States, although not as prolifically as in South America. In Japan, the commercial name of the mushroom is *Himematsutake;* its common name is *Kawariharatake*. It is also known by these names: Murrill's agaricus, Royal sun agaricus, and, less frequently, by its Chinese name *gee song rong* and almond-flavored portobello.

But the mushroom has the regrettable tendency to concentrate certain heavy metals, of which cadmium is the most dangerous. The amount of this toxic metal in Brazilian cultivars generally remained well below the legal limits. The same can be said about the mercury and lead content. However, some consignments of dried *Agaricus blazei* from China were found to contain excessive amounts of cadmium, although the mercury, lead, and arsenic concentrations were quite acceptable. I would certainly recommend to look for U.S.-cultivated, preferably organic types.

CULTIVATING *AGARICUS BLAZEI*

Attempts to cultivate *Agaricus blazei* with biotechnological assistance did not begin producing stable yields until the 1990s. *Agaricus blazei's* native tropical environment is very difficult to replicate. The mushroom is now being cultivated in Japan, Korea, the United States, Denmark, Holland, and Brazil. A few years ago, when the demand for *Agaricus blazei* skyrocketed and its price rose accordingly, the mushroom all but disappeared from the Piedade region of Brazil, according to some reports. But recently the taxonomy (identity) of this mushroom has been revised: the species grown in China, Japan, and Brazil is not *Agaricus blazei* but a new species now called *Agaricus brasiliensis*, or "the Brazilian *blazei*."

RESEARCH STUDIES OF *AGARICUS BLAZEI*

Clinical interest in *Agaricus blazei* began in earnest when a study showing antitumor activity by the mushroom was presented at a convention of the Japanese Cancer Association in 1980. In the study, *Agaricus blazei* was reported to have higher levels of beta-glucan than maitake, shiitake, or reishi mushrooms.

Beta-glucans are a kind of polysaccharide chain molecule that is found in medicinal mushrooms. Beta-glucans are known to help make the immune system more alert and balanced. Some scientists believe that *Agaricus blazei* contains the highest level of beta-glucans of any mushroom. They are (1-6)-(1-3)-beta-D-glucans, (1-6)-(1-4)-beta-D-glucans, polysaccharide-protein complex, RNA-protein complexes, and glucomannan. Many studies seem to show that the beta-glucans in *Agaricus blazei* are especially advantageous against tumor cells. Due to their low molecular weight, beta-glucans from *Agaricus blazei* can be absorbed into the body more easily than beta-glucans from other mushrooms, and this is believed to make them more effective. In 1995, Dr. Takashi Mizuno, who has studied *Agaricus blazei* for many years, stated that a beta-glucan he isolated in the mushroom was "the first case of an antitumor compound found in an edible mushroom."

The following are recent studies concerning the medicinal qualities of the mushroom.

Agaricus blazei and Cancer

Cancer is a complex immune-associated disease that can affect any organ or system of the body. It is caused by uncontrolled cell growth resulting from a genetic defect or cellular damage due to radiation or toxins in the environment. Although many advances have been made in the field of cancer research, there is still much to be done. Unfortunately, treatments such as radiation and chemotherapy can be as debilitating to the patients as the cancer itseif. Research indicates that conventional therapy used in combination with alternative therapies may help cancer patients.

Scientists at Kobe Pharmaceutical University, in Japan, tested the effects of *Agaricus blazei* on cancer. They injected a water-soluble fraction from *Agaricus blazei* into one group of cancerous mice and a saline solution into another group. Results of the experiment showed an increase in lymphocyte T cells, the immune system cells that are involved in protecting humans against cancer, in the *Agaricus blazei* group. The scientists concluded that beta-glucan from *Agaricus blazei* may be an effective preventative against cancer.

To immobilize or neutralize a malignant cell is not enough—the body needs to rid itself of the cell by making it burst and killing it. One way that the body destroys cells is by way of complement, a series of proteins that are produced in the liver. The activation of the complement cascade causes holes to be punched in the membrane of the targeted cell and its inside to

ooze out. The most active component of complement is called C3. Complement also attracts and stimulates macrophages to eat the malignant cells.
Recently, scientists at Mie University School of Medicine, in Japan, conducted experiments to gauge the effect of *Agaricus blazei* on complement
proteins made in the liver, specifically, the activity of the C3 complement.
The scientists implanted sarcoma tumors in mice and fed the mice a polysaccharide that they cultured from the mycelia of *Agaricus blazei*. The polysaccharide succeeded in stimulating macrophages in the mice and
activating C3 protein. From this, the scientists concluded that *Agaricus blazei*
could well be an aid in fighting the spread of malignant cancer cells in the
body.

Agaricus blazei and Tumors

Some herbal extracts, including those from mushrooms, are known to
attack tumors without doing any damage to normal tissue. In 1999, a group
of scientists from Japan extracted substances from *Agaricus blazei* in order
to monitor their effect on tumors in laboratory mice. The scientists injected
the tumor with the *Agaricus blazei* substances and noticed a marked inhibition in the tumor in the right flank, where they made the injection, and in
the left flank as well. One of the components of *the Agaricus blazei* extract
was a polysaccharide complex with a low molecular weight called alpha-
1,4-glucan-beta,-6-glucan. The scientists reported that this polysaccharide
had the strongest antitumor effect and was able to selectively kill tumor
cells without affecting normal cells.

Interestingly, the experiment also showed the possible activation of
granulocytes, which contain granules with potent chemicals that kill
microorganisms and play a role in controlling acute inflammatory reactions. The scientists speculated that both flanks of the tumor were inhibited because the granulocytes were able to migrate to the left flank of the
tumor. It seems that the *Agaricus blazei* polysaccharide examined in the
study not only inhibits tumors from growing, but it also stimulates the
migration of white blood cells that scavenge and kill malignant cells.

The same group of Japanese scientists conducted a similar experiment
with *Agaricus blazei* extracts. This time, the noninjected side of the tumor
also regressed, but the scientists noted that it regressed due to the activation of natural killer cells. What's more, the extract induced apoptosis (programmed cell death) in the malignant cells. Again, in this experiment, the
scientists observed that the *Agaricus blazei* extract killed tumor cells, but not

healthy cells. Then, the spleens of the treated mice were ground and dried and administered to a new generation of mice that were not given any *Agaricus blazei,* and the second group also showed around 80% rejection of implanted sarcoma tumors.

Research on *Agaricus blazei* beta-glucans is very active. Another anti-tumor substance from this unique mushroom is sodium pyroglutamate, which works in cutting off the blood supply to tumors. Recently, ergosterol, the biological precursor to vitamin D2, was found to be an active inhibitor of the growth of blood vessels required to nourish tumors (inhibition of angiogenesis), and the ergosterol of *Agaricus blazei* is a very active anti-angiogenic substance.

Other Benefits of *Agaricus blazei*

Agaricus blazei contains digestive enzymes such as amylase (which digests starches) and trypsin and other proteases (which digest meat). It also contains tyrosinase, which produces melanin, and has a hypotensive effect. The beta-glucans and oligosaccharides have demonstrated anti-hyperglycemic (anti-diabetic), anti-hypertriglyceridemic (lowering blood fat), anti-hyper-cholesterolemic (lowering cholesterol), and anti-arteriosclerotic (keeping the arteries flexible and young) activity. These findings are most important for diabetic patients.

Researchers at the Anti-Cancer Research Center of Japan treated 10 patients severely affected with chronic hepatitis with *Agaricus blazei.* The treatment proved "especially effective" in two patients, and effective in the other eight, in lowering elevated liver enzymes, serum globulins, and bile salts.

Very recent studies conducted in Oslo, Norway, have demonstrated activity of *Agaricus blazei* on cells of the immune system, the monocytes. These preliminary findings may indicate a potential use for *Agaricus blazei* in treating inflammatory and allergic conditions.

9

Phellinus linteus

ntil quite recently, *Phellinus linteus* was almost unknown outside the Korean peninsula. The mushroom is a relative newcomer and a rising superstar. For several hundred years, Korean physicians have prescribed *Phellinus linteus* as a treatment for cancer, stomach ailments, and arthritis. In traditional Korean medicine, the mushroom is known to ease pain caused by inflammation, and one medical text recommends it as a means of treating a red nose brought about by the immoderate drinking of alcohol. According to an old Korean saying, if you are able to find a yellow lump that grows on a mulberry tree, then you can bring a dying person back to life!

News of the mushroom's medicinal properties began reaching the outside world in the 1970s, when studies concerning *Phellinus linteus* were published in the Japanese and Chinese scientific press. In the past decade, manufacturers of Korean health-food products have marketed the mushroom aggressively, so convinced are they of its medicinal benefits. Reports about the mushroom's value as a treatment for arthritis have been circulating among herbalists in the United States and Europe for some time.

The etymology of the mushroom's Latin name is as follows: *Phellinus* means "cork" and *linteus* means "linen cloth." It is known as *"San-hwang"* in Korean, *"Mesimakobu"* in Japanese, and mulberry yellow polypore in the United States. Traditionally, the mushroom is boiled in water and is taken as a tea. Koreans sometimes soak it in wine or whisky before drinking it. *Phellinus linteus* is used as an ingredient in skin creams because it is believed to rejuvenate the skin.

An interesting sidelight of *Phellinus linteus* is the mushroom's part in bringing together scientific and commercial interests from North and South Korea. The governments of those nations, not known for cooperating with

Phellinus linteus

Until quite recently, *Phellinus linteus* was almost unknown outside the Korean peninsula. For several hundred years, Korean physicians have prescribed *Phellinus linteus* as a treatment for cancer, stomach ailments, and arthritis.

- Name: In Latin, *Phellinus* means "cork" and *linteus* means "linen cloth."

- Description: A thick, hard, woody, hoof-shaped mushroom with a bitter taste; it has a pale brown to light yellow cap; the stem is thick and varies in color from dark brown to black.

- Habitat: The mushroom favors dead or dying mulberry trees and is found in Korea and adjacent parts of China.

- Active ingredients: Polysaccharides (beta-glucans); proteoglycans.

- Uses: Powerful immunostimulant; anti-cancer (metastasis); antibacterial including antibiotic-resistant *Staphylococcus aureus;* anti-inflammatory and anti-arthritic; whitens skin.

one another, have permitted teams of scientists from both nations to conduct joint research. South Korea's Unification Ministry has permitted some business concerns from the south to import *Phellinus linteus* mushrooms from the north. Perhaps the healing properties of the mushroom touch the political as well as the biological realm.

PHELLINUS LINTEUS IN THE WILD

Phellinus linteus is a thick, hard, woody, hoof-shaped mushroom with a bitter taste. It has a pale brown to light yellow cap. The stem is thick and varies in color from dark brown to black. The mushroom favors dead or dying mulberry trees and is found in Korea and adjacent parts of China.

RESEARCH STUDIES OF *PHELLINUS LINTEUS*

Mushroom polysaccharides help awaken the immune system and keep it alert. One of the most interesting questions facing scientists who investigate the medicinal qualities of mushrooms is how the beta-glucans from the different mushrooms enhance the immune system differently. In 1999, scientists in Korea conducted an experiment to compare the activity of beta-glucan from *Phellinus linteus* with beta-glucan from *Basidiomycete* fungi. They conducted the tests both on laboratory mice and in culture. The scientists found the following in regard to *Phellinus linteus:*

- Increased activity by T lymphocytes and cytotoxic T cells, the white blood cells that destroy viruses and cells that have been mutated by cancer.

- Increased activity by natural killer cells and macrophages.

- Stimulation of the production of B cells, which in turn produce more antibodies to combat disease.

Phellinus linteus appears to exhibit a wider range of immunostimulation than other mushroom polysaccharides. It stimulates both the cell-mediated (macrophages, lymphocytes, natural killer cells, and so on) and the humoral (mediated by antibodies) parts of the immune system, proving that the mushroom is indeed a potent one.

Studies on *Phellinus linteus* are few and far between because the mushroom is a relative newcomer. Still, a few interesting studies have been presented in recent years.

Phellinus linteus, Tumors, and Metastasis

Recently, scientists in South Korea decided to see if *Phellinus linteus* could work alongside adriamycin, a popular chemotherapy drug, to inhibit tumors. They were especially interested in metastasis, the movement of tumor growth from one location in the body to another by way of blood circulation or the lymphatic system. The scientists wanted to see if *Phellinus linteus* in combination with adriamycin could inhibit metastasis. For the experiment, they implanted melanoma tumors in laboratory mice. They fed one group of mice *Phellinus linteus* and adriamycin, one group *Phellinus linteus* alone, and one group adriamycin alone. Then, the scientists looked at the growth of tumors in the mice, their survival rate, and the frequency of metastases in their lungs. Here are some of the findings of their study:

- Mice who took *Phellinus linteus* alone had a higher survival rate. In this group, tumor growth was inhibited and the frequency of metastases was reduced.

- In mice who took adriamycin alone, tumor growth was significantly inhibited, but metastasis was only slightly inhibited.

• The combination *of Phellinus linteus* and adriamycin was effective in inhibiting tumor growth, but not in inhibiting metastasis.

The scientists concluded that *Phellinus linteus* might be of use in conjunction with chemotherapy drugs such as adriamycin. Although *Phellinus linteus* doesn't work directly to kill cancer cells, it does help the immune system work better. Therefore, the mushroom might be useful as an adjunct to chemotherapy and other anticancer treatments.

It is also likely that anti-angiogenic activity of *Phellinus linteus*, as reported in 2004 by researchers from Sookmyung Women's University, in Korea, accounted for these results. *Phellinus linteus* subfractions specifically starve the blood supply of tumors and cancer metastases. Urologists of Gunma University School of Medicine, in Japan, described in 2004 a hormone refractory prostate cancer patient, with rapidly progressive bone metastasis, who showed dramatic response to intake of an extract of *Phellinus linteus*.

The Website of the Democratic People's Republic of Korea (a.k.a., North Korea) presents a table summarizing clinical results observed in 50 patients with diverse malignancies (liver, stomach, lung, colon, larynx, breast, and cervical cancers, as well as lymphoma). After 6 to 12 months, all patients reported an increase in appetite, general well-being, and reduction (or even control) of pain; the patients with cancer of the stomach gained weight. (Obviously, these results must be considered according to their source.)

Other Benefits of *Phellinus linteus*

The extract of *Phellinus linteus* grown on germinated brown rice modulated the production of IgE, the antibody associated with allergic conditions, and the ratio of Th1/Th2 cytokine secretion that is considered as critical in the development of allergic disease. *Phellinus linteus* extract may prove important in preventing the current spread of allergies and asthma.

It is also a potent antibacterial against the menacing methicillin-resistant *Staphylococcus aureus* (MRSA) bacteria that are the scourge of hospitals and patients with a weakened immune system. Alcoholic extracts and a proteoglycan from *Phellinus linteus* show an anti-inflammatory effect in the collagen-induced arthritis and in the croton oil-induced ear edema test in mice, and could possibly be a new nonsteroidal anti-inflammatory.

10

Trametes versicolor

rametes versicolor has the distinction of being the mushroom from which one of the world's leading anticancer drugs, Krestin, is derived. Although Krestin has not been approved for use by the United States Food and Drug Administration (FDA), it was the best-selling anticancer drug in Japan for much of the 1980s. Krestin was the first mushroom-derived anticancer drug to be approved by the Japanese government's Health and Welfare Ministry, the equivalent of the FDA. All health-care plans in Japan cover members' purchases of Krestin.

The Latin etymology of *Trametes versicolor* is as follows: *Trametes* means "one who is thin" and *versicolor* means "variously colored." In some literature, the mushroom is called *Coriolus versicolor* or, rarely, *Polyporus versicolor,* but taxonomists now agree that the mushroom should properly be classified *Trametes.* In China, the mushroom is called *yun zhi,* or "cloud mushroom." In Japan, it is called *Kawaratake,* which means "beside-the-river mushroom."

TRAMETES VERSICOLOR IN THE WILD

Trametes versicolor is found in temperate forests throughout the world and in all of the United States. It is lovely and is occasionally included in floral displays. In the English-speaking world, the mushroom is known as the "Turkey Tail" because its fan shape resembles the tail of a standing turkey. It is striped with dark-to-light brown bands that alternate with bands of orange, blue, white, and tan. It prefers to grow on dead logs and has been known to feed on most kinds of trees.

The Japanese have long used *Trametes versicolor* as a folk remedy for cancer. In traditional Chinese medicine, *Trametes versicolor* is used to treat

Trametes versicolor

Trametes versicolor has the distinction of being the mushroom from which one of the world's leading anticancer drugs, Krestin, is derived.

• Name: In Latin, *Trametes* means "one who is thin" and *versicolor* means "variously colored." Other names include "cloud mushroom," "beside-the-river mushroom," and "Turkey Tail." In Chinese, it is known as *yun zhi.*

• Description: It is striped with dark-to-light brown bands that alternate with bands of orange, blue, white, and tan.

• Habitat: Found in temperate forests throughout the world and in all of the United States. It prefers to grow on dead logs and has been known to feed on most kinds of trees.

• Active ingredients: Polysaccharide-K (1-3 beta-glucan); polysaccharide-peptide.

• Uses: Immunostimulant; anti-cancer (lung, stomach, esophagus); lowers LDL ("bad") cholesterol; antiviral (HIV, cytomegalovirus); controls septic shock.

---

lung infections, excess phlegm, and hepatitis. The ancient Taoists revered the mushroom because it grows on pine trees. Because pines are evergreens, Taoist priests assumed that the mushroom had the staying power of the pine tree, which never loses its foliage. Taoists believed that *Trametes versicolor* collects *yang* energy from the roots of the pine tree, and they prescribed it for patients whose *yang* energy was deficient.

RESEARCH STUDIES ON *TRAMETES VERSICOLOR*

Trametes versicolor came to the attention of the pharmaceutical industry in 1965 when a chemical engineer working for Kureha Chemical Industry Company Ltd., in Japan, observed his neighbor attempting to cure himself of gastric cancer with a folk remedy. The neighbor was in the late stages of cancer and had been rejected for treatment by hospitals and clinics. For several months, he took the folk remedy, a mushroom, and then, having been cured, he went back to work. The folk remedy was *Trametes versicolor.*

The engineer convinced his colleagues to examine the mushroom. The best strain of *Trametes versicolor* was found and cultivated. Soon PSK, an extract from the mushroom, was born. PSK (Polysaccharide-K) is the chief ingredient in Krestin: it is 1-3 beta-glucan, the type of polysaccharide found in medicinal mushrooms; but it is bound to a protein and is especially beneficial to the immune system.

The success of Krestin inspired Chinese researchers to develop a *Trametes versicolor* extract of their own called PSP (Polysaccharide-Peptide). A peptide is a compound of low molecular weight that figures in the creation of proteins. Both PSK and PSP are potent immunostimulators with specific activity for T cells and for antigen-presenting cells such as monocytes and macrophages. The biologic activity is characterized by their ability to increase white blood cell counts, interferon-alpha and interleukin-2 production, and delayed-type hypersensitivity reactions. Clinical experimentation with PSP did not begin until the early 1990s, whereas clinical studies of PSK have been conducted since 1978. At the 14th annual International Chemotherapy Symposium in 1991, 68 papers about PSK were presented, about one-fifth of all papers.

Krestin, PSK, and Cancer

PSK is extracted from a mycelial strain CM-101 and is approximately 62% polysaccharide and 38% protein. The glucan portion of PSK consists of a beta 1-4 main chain and beta 1-3 side chain, with beta 1-6 side chains. The polypeptide portion is rich in aspartic, glutamic, and other amino acids and is orally bioavailable. PSK has been shown to have no substantial effect on immune responses of the host under normal conditions. It can restore the immune potential to the normal level after the host was depressed by tumor burden or anticancer chemotherapeutic agents. This compound has been systematically tested against a wide range of human cancers with some considerable success.

After intra-tumoral administration, PSK causes local inflammatory responses that result in the nonspecific killing of these abnormal cells. Consequently, local administration of PSK is more efficient than systemic use. It has been reported that PSK induces gene expression of some cytokines such as TNF-alpha, interleukin (IL)-1, IL-8, and IL-6. These cytokines, produced by monocytes, macrophages, and various other cell types, directly stimulate cytotoxic T cells against tumors, enhance antibody production by B lymphocytes, and induce IL-2 receptor expression on T lymphocytes. Interestingly, recent studies indicate that PSK exerts tumoricidal activity by inducing T cells that recognize PSK as an antigen and kill tumor cells in an antigen-specific manner.

The drug is almost always prescribed to cancer patients who have had a tumor removed and are undergoing chemotherapy or radiotherapy. It is often prescribed for colon, lung, stomach, and esophageal cancer and has no side effects. Here are recent studies that demonstrate the effectiveness of PSK on cancer patients' immune systems:

- In a 10-year study of 185 lung cancer patients who were undergoing radiotherapy, Japanese doctors administered Krestin to roughly half the patients (the others got a placebo). The idea was to see whether Krestin could boost the cancer patients' white blood cell activity and thereby strengthen their immune systems. After 10 years, 39% of patients who had Stage I or II lung cancer and took Krestin survived, while only 16% survived in the non-Krestin group. Of Stage III cancer patients, 22% survived in the Krestin group, but only 5% of the patients who did not take Krestin survived.

  In a randomized, controlled clinical trial of 227 patients with breast cancer, doctors prescribed PSK and chemotherapy for some patients and chemotherapy alone for others. In this 10-year study, 81.1% of patients who took PSK and were treated with chemotherapy survived, while 64.5% of patients who had chemotherapy alone survived. Early studies with breast cancer patients seemed to imply that long-term PSK immunotherapy in conjunction with chemotherapy could have beneficial results. In a later, much larger trial (914 patients), in-depth analysis implied that PSK significantly extended survival in ER-negative, Stage II patients without lymph node involvement. However, in a further large trial, researchers could find no statistical evidence of any benefit from PSK.

  These contradictory studies may have been clarified by researchers who compared patients who were positive for HLA-B40 antigen (a surface cell marker) treated with PSK against patients who were B40 negatives. It was found that B40-positive patients treated with PSK (3 g daily, for a two-month course each year) in addition to chemotherapy had an improved 10-year overall survival rate compared to B40-negative patients. Thus, HLA-B40 may be a predictive factor for PSK response.

- In a five-year study of 262 stomach cancer patients who had gastrectomies (a removal of part of the stomach), some patients received PSK along with their chemotherapy treatment and some did not. Of the patients who received PSK, 73% were still living after five years; the survival rate of the other group was 60%. The study concluded that PSK along with chemotherapy was "beneficial for preventing recurrence of

cancer and in prolonging survival for patients who have undergone curative gastrectomy." Researchers had previously observed that dendritic
cells could infiltrate gastric cancers in some patients, which correlated
with an increase in disease-free and overall survival post-surgery. It was
concluded that patients with gastric cancer with limited dendritic cell
infiltration prior to surgery were more likely to have significant response
when given PSK immunotherapy. The most recent trial of PSK in the
treatment of gastric cancer carried out in Japan showed that combining
PSK with conventional chemotherapy significantly improved overall
survival.

- In another, more recent study, PSK improved overall survival in
  esophageal cancer in patients with levels of pre-operative high beta-1-
  antichymotrypsin or sialic acid.

- In a study of 185 patients with epidermoid carcinoma, adenocarcinoma,
  or large-cell carcinoma given PSK as an immune system potentiator following radiotherapy, almost four times more patients who were treated
  with PSK had significant improvements in disease-free survival than
  those not given PSK. PSK was clinically significant with more advanced
  patients (Stage III disease) than Stage I and II patients. PSK had greater
  activity for older patients (over 70 years) and patients with small primary tumors.

Krestin came under fire beginning in the late 1980s at several medical
conventions, where doctors questioned its effectiveness. The substance, it
seemed, had been overhyped. The Health and Welfare Ministry in Japan
now instructs doctors to use Krestin only as an adjunct to chemotherapy or
radiotherapy. The drug by itself is not supposed to be used as a treatment
for cancer. PSK can raise survival rates in cancer patients and prolong their
lives. Moreover, the substance is nontoxic. Because the risk to patients of
taking PSK appears minimal and the rewards are many, PSK is likely to be
an aid in fighting cancer for years to come. PSK also causes decreases in
LDL ("bad") cholesterol in patients with high levels of blood circulating
fat. It was found to have an antiviral effect on HIV and cytomegalovirus.

PSP and Cancer

PSP was first isolated from cultured deep-layer mycelium of the COV-1
strain of *Trametes versicolor* in 1983. PSP may contain at least four discrete
molecules, all of which are true proteoglycans. PSP differs from PSK in its

saccharide makeup, lacking fucose and containing arabinose and rhamnose. The polysaccharide chains are true beta-glucans, mainly 1-4, 1-2 and 1-3 glucose linkages with small amounts of galactose, mannose, and arabinose linkages. PSP can be easily delivered by oral route.

Like PSK, PSP is prescribed to cancer patients to help improve their immune systems before and after surgical treatment, chemotherapy, and radiotherapy. China's Ministry of Public Health approved PSP as a national class I medical material in 1992. In 1999, PSP was added to the list of medicines whose cost could be reimbursed by medical insurance programs. What's more, the National Cancer Research Center in the United States has declared PSP a fungous anticancerous substance. The PSP that has been researched here is derived from a special strain of *Trametes versicolor* called COV-1 developed in China. Here are recent studies concerning PSP:

- Scientists at the University of Shanghai studied 650 cancer patients who were undergoing chemotherapy or radiotherapy to see if PSP could ameliorate the side effects of treatment. Using 20 criteria for assessing adverse reactions to anticancer drugs (weakness, night sweats, and others), the scientists determined that the PSP group had markedly fewer side effects than the control group.

- In a placebo-controlled study, researchers at the Shanghai Institute of Chinese Medicine administered PSP to one group undergoing chemotherapy or radiotherapy for cancer and a placebo to another group. Then, they observed both groups for evidence of anorexia, vomiting, dry throat, and other side effects, as well as increased weight, higher natural killer cell counts, and other signs of improvement. What the researchers called "the overall effective rate" (the rate at which patients' health improved) was significantly higher in the PSP group (85.8%) than the control group (41.9%).

There is a dramatic anti-tumor effect when PSP is combined with interleukin-2 (IL-2). As side effects of IL-2 are dose-dependent, it is reasonable to expect that with PSP, a lower dose of IL-2 could be used clinically with subsequent decrease in the severity of the side effects. PSP in combination with radiotherapy induced a significant increase in the percentage of apoptotic cells (i.e., cells "committing suicide") at 24 hours, compared with radiation alone, and it has been surmised that the antitumor mechanism of PSP may also involve the induction of DNA damage by apoptosis in the target cancer cells.

- A common adverse reaction of radiotherapy and chemotherapy is hematopoietic toxicity in the bone marrow, resulting in anemia and increased susceptibility to infections. Several studies have shown a strong amelioration of these toxic effects by PSP.

- In a double-blind, placebo-controlled randomized study, physicians at the Queen Mary Hospital of the University of Hong Kong evaluated the effects of a 28-day administration of PSP on patients who had completed conventional treatment for advanced non-small cell lung cancer (NSCLC), a very aggressive form of lung cancer. Thirty-four patients, with no significant difference in their baseline demographic, clinical, or tumor characteristics, or previous treatment regimens, were enrolled into each of the PSP and placebo groups. After 28 days of treatment, there was a significant improvement in the number of white blood cells, including neutrophils and immunoglobulins G and M, and percent of body fat among the PSP-treated patients, but not the placebo-treated patients; this difference was statistically very significant. Although the evaluable PSP patients did not improve in NSCLC-related symptoms, there were significantly less PSP patients withdrawn due to disease progression than their control counterparts: 5.9% and 23.5%, respectively. There was no reported adverse reaction attributable to PSP. Researchers concluded that PSP treatment appeared to be associated with slower deterioration in patients with advanced non-small cell lung cancer.

- PSP stimulates lymphokine-activated-killer (LAK) cell proliferation, and reduces the concentration of IL-2 needed to produce a cytotoxic response. PSP (2 g/kg per day) possesses immunopotentiating activities, effective in restoring clinically induced immunosuppression, such as depressed lymphocyte proliferation, NK cell function, production of white blood cells. and the growth of spleen and thymus in rats. In addition, PSP increased both IgG and IL-2 production.

  PSP is safe. A series of recent extensive series of experiments on possible genetic toxicity of the PSP polysaccharopeptide found no evidence of mutagenic or toxic effects. Subchronic toxicity tests have been performed with various concentrations of PSP on rats by oral administration and no obvious effects were observed.

Trametes versicolor and Septic Shock

Septic shock is a complex syndrome mediated by binding of lipopolysaccharide (LPS) from gram-negative bacteria to immune cells and the following release of a cascade of inflammatory mediators and reactive oxygen species. Because of the large number of patients with septic shock, a great deal of effort is necessary to develop new therapeutic possibilities. Extracts of the fruiting bodies of *Trametes versicolor* inhibit *in vitro* binding of LPS to the receptor and could therefore contain lead structures for drugs against LPS-mediated septic shock.

11

Hericium erinaceus

ericium erinaceus is found throughout the northern hemisphere in Europe, East Asia, and North America. The mushroom's exotic, other-worldly appearance has inspired admirers to give it a host of unusual names: Lion's Mane, Monkey's Mushroom, Monkey's Head, Bear's Head, Hog's Head Fungus, White Beard, Old Man's Beard, Bearded Hedgehog, Hedgehog Mushroom, Pom Pom (because it resembles the ornamental pom-pom ball on the end of a stocking cap), and Pom Pom Blanc (because *Hericium erinaceus* is white to off-white in color).

In Japan, the mushroom is known chiefly as *Yamabushitake*. *Yamabushi*, literally "those who sleep in the mountains," are hermit monks of the *Shugen-do* sect of ascetic Buddhism. *Hericium erinaceus* is supposed to resemble the *suzukake*, an ornamental garment that these monks wear. *Take* means "mushroom" in Japanese. In China, the mushroom goes by the name *shishigashira*, which means "lion's head," and *Houtou*, which means "baby monkey." In some literature, *Hericium erinaceus* is mistakenly called *Hericium erinaceum*.

In traditional Chinese medicine, *Hericium erinaceus* is prescribed for stomach disorders, ulcers, and gastrointestinal ailments. A powder extract from the mushroom called *Houtou* is sold in China. In North America, Native Americans used *Hericium erinaceus* as a styptic, applied as a dried powder to cuts and scratches to stop them from bleeding. The mushroom was commonly found in Native Americans' medicine bags.

Hericium erinaceus is a culinary as well as a medicinal mushroom. To some, it gives the hint of seafood, crab, or lobster flavor. The mushroom has a rubbery texture similar to squid. The commercial cultivation of *Hericium erinaceus* began quite recently. Until two decades ago, the mushroom was considered a rare find in the forest, but now its name can be found on the menus of gourmet restaurants.

Hericium erinaceus

In traditional Chinese medicine, *Hericium erinaceus* is prescribed for stomach disorders, ulcers, and gastrointestinal ailments. It is a culinary as well as a medicinal mushroom, giving a hint of seafood, crab, or lobster flavor.

• Name: In Japan, the mushroom is known as *Yamabushitake. Yamabushi,* literally "those who sleep in the mountains," are hermit monks and *Hericium erinaceus* is supposed to resemble the *suzukake,* an ornamental garment that these monks wear; *take* means "mushroom." In China, the mushroom goes by the name *shishigashira,* which means "lion's head," and *houtou,* which means "baby monkey." Also known as Lion's Mane, Monkey's Mushroom, Monkey's Head, Bear's Head, Hog's Head Fungus, White Beard, Old Man's Beard, Bearded Hedgehog, Hedgehog Mushroom, and Pom Pom.

• Description: The mushroom is 2–8 inches across. Its white, icicle-like tendrils hang from a rubbery base.

• Habitat: Found throughout the northern hemisphere in Europe, East Asia, and North America. The mushroom favors dead or dying broadleaf trees such as oak, walnut, and beech.

• Active ingredients: Polysaccharides; fatty acids (Y-A-2); hericenons A and B, and hericenons C, D, E, F, G, and H. The mycelium also contains a group of diterpenes called erinacines that mimic the nerve growth factor; one erinacine is an opioid (useful for pain control).

• Uses: Styptic; immunostimulant; anti-cancer (stomach, esophagus, skin); anti-sarcoma; helps control Alzheimer's disease; antioxidant; regulates glucose, triglycerides, and cholesterol (mostly LDL) blood levels.

HERICIUM ERINACEUS IN THE WILD

The mushroom is 2–8 inches across. Its white, icicle-like tendrils hang from a rubbery base. A sharp knife is often needed to remove the mushroom from the hardwood from which it grows. The mushroom favors dead or dying broadleaf trees such as oak, walnut, and beech. Recently, *Hericium erinaceus* was blamed in northern California for an outbreak of heart rot in live oak trees.

CULTIVATING *HERICIUM ERINACEUS*

Chinese pharmacies carry pills and powders that are made from *Hericium erinaceus*. Very likely the people who take these powders don't realize that they are taking powder cultivated with techniques developed in Sonoma County, California. How the *Hericium erinaceus* got from Sonoma County to China makes for an interesting story and it also illustrates how mycologists share information about medicinal mushrooms.

In 1980, a fellow mycologist informed Malcolm Clark that he had seen an unusual fruiting of *Hericium erinaceus* on a tree in Glen Ellen, a small town in Sonoma County, some 50 miles north of San Francisco. He was told that the *Hericium erinaceus* specimen grew on a bay tree that had fallen over a winter creek. Clark, seizing the opportunity to study *Hericium erinaceus* firsthand, took his sleeping bag and some instruments from his laboratory in Sonoma County to the site in Glen Ellen and camped there for three days.

"I just watched the thing for a while," he said. "I lived with it. It was important for me to be with the mushroom." Clark took observations regarding sun exposure, light, and humidity. He measured the mushroom. After the three days were over, he harvested the mushroom and took it back to his lab, where he cultured the *Hericium erinaceus* specimen. "I was able to make up a substrate and fruit the mushroom according to what I had been able to observe," he recounted. "Then it was a case of improving it to find out how much better I could make it grow and under what control conditions."

Clark's chief interest in *Hericium erinaceus* at this time was developing the mushroom for the culinary market. He took it to world-renowned Ernie's Restaurant in San Francisco, where chef Jacky Robert took one look at the mushroom in his hand and exclaimed, "Ah, Pom Pom Blanc." Clark trademarked the name and Pom Pom Blancs are now available in many gourmet restaurants.

RESEARCH STUDIES ON *HERICIUM ERINACEUS*

Western science opened the book on *Hericium erinaceus* a few short years ago. Although the mushroom has been part of the diet in Japan and China for many centuries and its medicinal properties as a styptic are well known, scientists have hardly begun to study it. However, the mushroom has turned a few heads for its unusual medicinal properties. In a recent article in the *International Journal of Medicinal Mushrooms*, Dr. Takashi Mizuno of Shizouka University, in Japan, noted the following about *Hericium erinaceus*:

• Owing to their effect on the immune system, polysaccharides from the fruit-body of the mushroom may help against stomach, esophageal, and skin cancer. These polysaccharides modulate the immune system so that it responds more effectively and helps people who have cancer to control the disease and manage the side effects of chemotherapy.

• Preliminary studies show that low-molecular-weight constituents such as phenols (hercenon A and B) and fatty acids (Y-A-2) from *Hericium erinaceus* may have chemotherapeutic effects on cancer. These molecules seem to operate directly against cancer cells.

Hericium erinaceus and Alzheimer's Disease

What was especially intriguing about Takashi Mizuno's article was its implications for the treatment of Alzheimer's disease. Some 4 million Americans suffer from this affliction, the most common form of irreversible dementia. Symptoms of Alzheimer's disease include confusion, memory loss, disorientation, and the inability to speak or reason. Scientists believe that the disease is caused in the brain by plaque buildup around nerve cells and by distorted nerve fibers called neurofibrillary tangles. Alzheimer's disease has no known cure, and it is always fatal.

Dr. Mizuno reported that compounds in *Hericium erinaceus* (hericenons C, D, E, F, G, H) may encourage the production of a protein called nerve growth factor (NGF), which is required in the brain for developing and maintaining important sensory neurons. To put it simply, *Hericium erinaceus* may regenerate nerve tissue in the brain. This might have an ameliorative effect in Alzheimer's dementia, a unique opportunity that is actively studied in Japan, a country with a large aging population.

Hericium erinaceus and Cholesterol and Diabetes

Recent studies have shown that *Hericium erinaceus* extracts have antioxidant activities, regulate the levels of blood lipids (fats), and reduce blood glucose levels. In diabetic rats, the effects on blood glucose, serum triglyceride, and total cholesterol levels were very significant in the rats fed daily with a concentrate of *Hericium erinaceus* at 1g/kg body weight. The exo-biopolymer produced from a submerged mycelium culture of *Hericium erinaceus* was even much more active, at a dose of 200 mg/kg body weight, in reducing plasma total cholesterol (32.9%), LDL ("bad") cholesterol (45.4%), triglyceride (34.3%), atherogenic index (58.7%), and the activity of the hepatic enzyme HMG-CoA reductase (20.2%).

Hericium erinaceus and the Immune System

Recently, scientists at Zhejiang College of Traditional Chinese Medicine, in Hangzhou, China, undertook an experiment to find out whether *Hericium erinaceus* can activate T and B lymphocytes in the immune system. These white blood cells circulate in the lymph and blood and flush viruses and bacteria from the body. The scientists were interested in knowing how *Hericium erinaceus* affected the lymphocytes and what would happen if the mushroom were used in conjunction with other substances known to stimulate lymphocyte production.

The scientists isolated T and B lymphocytes from the blood of laboratory mice. They placed the lymphocytes in test tubes and spiked the test tubes with various combinations of a lectin called Con-A, polysaccharides from *Hericium erinaceus,* and lipopolysaccharide (LPS), another stimulant of white blood cells. The scientists observed the following:

- *Hericium erinaceus* polysaccharides and Con-A together made the T lymphocytes proliferate at three times the rate they proliferated when Con-A alone was used. *Hericium erinaceus* alone, without Con-A, had no effect on lymphocytes.

- *Hericium erinaceus* polysaccharides and LPS together made lymphocytes proliferate at two to three times the rate they proliferate with LPS alone. Once again, *Hericium erinaceus* polysaccharides alone had no effect on lymphocyte production.

From this experiment, it appears that *Hericium erinaceus* can play a role in boosting the immune system when it is used in combination with other substances, namely Con-A and lipopolysaccharide (LPS). In another recent experiment conducted at the Tajen Institute of Technology, in Taiwan, water-soluble polysaccharides of *Hericium erinaceus* increased significantly the number of CD4+ cells and macrophages in mice, when compared to a control group.

Hericium erinaceus and Sarcoma Tumors

To test the effectiveness of *Hericium erinaceus* on tumors, scientists at the Kyoritsu Pharmaceutical and Industrial Company, in Japan, transplanted sarcoma tumors into laboratory mice and fed the mice different doses of dried mushroom powder for 14 days. At the end of the period, they cut out the tumors and weighed them to see if they had grown. The result of their experiment: the tumors either shrank or stopped growing.

The interesting aspect of this experiment, however, had to do with the mushroom's overall effect on the immune system. The scientists concluded that T cells had not shrunk the tumors. *Hericium erinaceus* is not chemotherapeutic. The *Hericium erinaceus* extract worked by stimulating the immune system of the animal, which in turn helped to control and reduce the burden of the sarcoma tumor.

12

Miscellaneous Mushrooms

A number of other mushroom varieties are showing great promise as medicinals, and although research is limited, the science is confirming their healing potential. Here, we cover a few of these relatively unknown fungi.

AGARICUS BISPORUS

Agaricus bisporus is the interesting name for this mushroom. An apparently older name for this mushroom is *Agaricus brunnescens*, referring to the oxidative "browning" reaction when the mushroom is bruised. *Agaricus,* cleverly, means gilled mushroom. In the early days of mycology, the study of mushrooms, every gilled mushroom was placed in the genus *Agaricus.* Now, *Agaricus* is restricted to saprophytic mushrooms with a chocolate brown spore print and usually an annulus (ring) around the stalk. *Bisporus* refers to the two-spored basidia lining the gills; these spores are shed separately and must find a mate in order to form mushrooms again. Each of the spores on *Agaricus* already contains the nuclei needed for sexual reproduction and does not need to find a mate. This ensures that every spore that lands on a suitable substrate is capable of forming mushrooms.

Agaricus bisporus is the most commonly grown mushroom in the United States, accounting for up to 90% of the mushroom production. However, *Agaricus* accounts for less than 40% of worldwide production. *Agaricus bisporus* has increased in popularity in North America with the introduction of two brown strains, portobello and crimini. Portobello is a marketing name for more flavorful brown strains of *Agaricus bisporus* that are allowed to open to expose the mature gills with brown spores; crimini is the same brown strain but it is not allowed to open before harvesting. Per capita consumption of fresh *Agaricus* in the United States is about 2.2 pounds (1 kilo-gram) per year.

There are many other species of *Agaricus*. In some parts of the U.S., *Agaricus bitorquis,* the "double ring *Agaricus*," is rather common and abundant and has a much stronger flavor than cultivated *A. bisporus.* "The Prince," *A. augustus,* is a rather large mushroom that is more common in western North America and has a pleasant almond flavor. *A. campestris* is known as the "meadow mushroom"; it is the most closely related wild relative of *A. bisporus.* The "horse mushroom," *A. arvensis,* is also excellent. The edible wild *Agaricus* varieties have mostly strong and delicious flavors, ranging from a stronger version of the white button to some that are even almondy in smell and flavor. *Agaricus bisporus,* though not as distinctive as other *Agaricus* species, can be recognized by the following characteristics: relatively short stature, a cap with pale brown scales, flesh that bruises slowly to reddish-brown, a well-developed ring, smooth stipe, and a preference for fruiting with Monterey cypress.

Recent scientific studies of *Agaricus* have focused on cancer and prevention of blindness. A lectin from *Agaricus bisporus* can help prevent the spread of human epithelial cancer cells, without being toxic to the body. This property confers to it an important therapeutic potential as an antineoplastic agent. Estrogen is a major factor in the development of breast cancer and plays a dominant role in tumor proliferation. Vegetables that contain certain phytochemicals can suppress breast cancer spread by inhibiting the enzyme aromatase/estrogen synthetase, which produces estrogen in the body. *Agaricus bisporus* extract suppressed aromatase activity dose dependently, suggesting that diets high in mushrooms may function in chemoprevention in postmenopausal women by reducing the *in situ* production of estrogen.

The lectin from *Agaricus bisporus* (ABL) has antiproliferative effects on a range of cell types. Researchers from Liverpool, England, tested whether it might inhibit Tenon's capsule fibroblasts in models of wound healing and therefore have a use in the modification of scar formation after glaucoma surgery. ABL caused a dose-dependent inhibition of proliferation and lattice contraction without significant toxicity. ABL might be especially useful where subtle modification of healing is needed, as in eye surgery for glaucoma.

Another group of ophthalmologists at the University of Liverpool studied the effects of ABL on the pigment epithelium of the retina. The retinal pigment epithelium (RPE) plays a major role in the development of proliferative vitreoretinopathy (PVR), a major cause of blindness. In particular,

RPE cells are implicated in generating the contraction forces seen. The study showed that ABL inhibits contraction and adhesion of human RPE cells *in vitro* without apparent cytotoxicity. *Agaricus,* therefore, deserves consideration as a potential therapeutic agent in the prevention and treatment of PVR and possibly other non-ocular wound-healing processes.

ANTRODIA CAMPHORATA

Antrodia camphorata is also called *niu zhang zhi* and red camphor mushroom and is a fungus unique to Taiwan. It grows inside the rotten heartwood of the camphor tree, *Cinnamomum kanehirai,* at a altitude of 1,350–6,000 feet. It has strong smell of yellow camphor and was primarily collected in the wild until very recently. Because this mushroom is rare, it is very expensive.

Recent studies of *Antrodia camphorata,* conducted at the National Taiwan University Graduate School of Pharmacy, Chinese Medical College, Southern Taiwan University of Technology, and others, found that it contains many active substances. Successful culture of the fruiting bodies found concentrations of diterpenes and triterpenes similar to the ones found in the rare wild mushroom. These had anti-inflammatory activities, major free-radical scavenging properties (antioxidants), and significant immunomodulating properties.

Antrodia camphorata extracts protect the liver against toxicity and liver fibrosis and they also demonstrate neuroprotective activities. The growth of a breast cancer cell line was inhibited by *Antrodia camphorata* extracts of fruiting bodies. The polysaccharides extracted from the fruiting bodies of *Antrodia camphorata* exhibit significant antiviral activity against the hepatitis B virus. And, finally, extracts from cultured mycelia of *Antrodia camphorata* display anti-inflammatory effects as well.

DICTYOPHORA INDUSIATA

Dictyophora indusiata (also known as "veiled lady mushroom" or basket stinkhorn) is a tropical stinkhorn fungus with a pale yellow, netlike veil (indusium) that hangs down from the cap (head). It is up to 7 inches tall, white and spongy, with a conical cap covered in a slimy, spore-bearing mass with the odor of rotting flesh. It comes out in the bamboo groves in the rainy season. Called net stinkhorn or bamboo fungus, the dried fungi are commonly sold in Asian markets. For cooking, the dried stinkhorns are hydrated and cooked in water, then simmered until tender.

Research has shown that several components of *Dictyophora indusiata* could protect or improve the central nervous system, while others are anti-inflammatory. Dictyoquinazols A, B, and C have been isolated from the extract of *Dictyophora indusiata*. Research has shown that dictyoquinazols protect primary cultured mouse cortical neurons from excitotoxicities in a dose-dependent manner. In addition, dictyophorines from *Dictyophora indusiata* promoted nerve growth factor (NGF) synthesis by astroglial cells. Finally, an extract of the fruit bodies of *Dictyophora indusita* exhibited anti-inflammatory effects on both edema and hyperalgesia in studies with rats.

FOMITOPSIS OFFICINALIS

The Greek physician Dioscorides included the larch polypore (*Fomitopsis officinalis*) in his *De Materia Medica*, published approximately 65 CE. Known then as *Agaricum* or *Agarikon,* and later as the quinine conk or brown trunk rot, it was used as a treatment for "consumption," a disease now known as tuberculosis. The *Agarikon* was a staple of pharmacology until at least the 18th century, when it fell into obscurity.

For hundreds of years, the Haida of the Queen Charlotte Islands of British Columbia and other coastal indigenous peoples have used shelf polypore fungi medicinally. The Haida gave *Fomitopsis officinalis* a name that translates into "ghost bread" or "tree biscuit." Shelf fungi were also used for spiritual practices and have been found in shaman's graves. The Haida even personified bracket fungus as "Fungus Man" in their mythology.

Fomitopsis officinalis grows on western larch, amabilis and grand fir, Engelmann and Sitka spruce, lodgepole, ponderosa, and western white pine, Douglas fir, and western hemlock. Elsewhere in North America, it has also been found on white and black spruce. It is extinct or nearly so in Europe and Asia. Fruiting bodies are formed relatively frequently on larch, but are less common on other species. On all hosts, a single fruiting body indicates that most of the wood volume has been destroyed.

The fruiting bodies are perennial and vary from hoof-shaped to long pendulous structures. They can grow up to 16 inches in diameter. The upper surface is zoned, white when fresh but drying to dark gray or light brown in old specimens; a chalky coating, which rubs off as a white powder, may be present. (The powder is used by the Cree Indians as a styptic to stop bleeding.) The lower surface is white when fresh, drying to light brown, and the pores are relatively small and uniform in outline. The context is white or gray, relatively soft when young, then toughening with age.

The bitter taste of the sporophore context and mycelial mats has given this fungus the common name "quinine fungus."

Recent tests demonstrate that a specially prepared extract from *Fomitopsis officinalis* is highly selective against viruses. A National Institutes of Health screening program tests mushroom extracts against viruses that could be weaponized, including the viruses causing yellow fever, dengue, SARS, respiratory viruses, and pox viruses. Several of the *Fomitopsis officinalis* samples showed activity for reducing infection from vaccinia and cowpox, both smallpox viruses. While several strains of extract generated strong anti-pox activity, other strains were less potent.

PORIA COCOS

Poria cocos is known in China as *fu ling* and is elsewhere called tuckahoe, Indian potato, or Hoelen. It grows on the roots of old, dead pine trees. Fu Ling's original name referred to the fact that this mushroom was lying on the ground (*fu*) and was thought to be the spirit (*ling*) of the pine tree. In the wild, *Poria cocos* grows like the truffle, only around the roots of certain pine trees instead of oaks. There is an interesting history of its use in North America: the Native Americans used it to make bread and European settlers observed them digging the mushrooms out of the ground; thus, the Europeans incorrectly called it "Indian potato." It later became a survival food for African slaves running to freedom and was called "tuckahoe" by them. Sometimes, a single *Poria cocos* mushroom could weigh as much as 15 to 30 pounds!

The form of *Poria* used as a medicinal grows as a subterranean mass of hardened mycelial tissue called sclerotia. *Poria* is composed mainly of polysaccharides and also contains some triterpenoids. Two of the polysaccharides are beta-pachyman and poriatin. Poriatin has been shown to increase the antitumor effects of some chemotherapeutic agents. Pachyman can be chemically converted to pachymaran, which shows a high degree of antitumor activity. Other constituents of *Poria cocos* include the polysaccharide beta-pachymarose, several organic acids (tumulosic acid, eubricoic acid, pinicolic acid, and pachymic acid), chitin, protein, sterols, lecithin, and choline.

Little Western research has been done with this mushroom. However, *Poria* is the most widely used fungus in traditional Chinese medicine (TCM) formulas. Traditionally used in China as a tonic soup for the elderly and infirm, *Poria cocos* is also given to children for growth and sustenance properties as well. In the TCM system, it is said to soothe the heart, strengthen vital energy, and calm agitation. One of the reasons *Poria cocos* is so highly valued is because the active compounds are extremely easy to digest and assimilate. It is used as a diuretic and a cure for edema, excess fluids which can cause swelling.

Traditional practitioners focused on the mushroom fruit body and the sclerotia, which were the only parts of the plant that could be harvested. A sclerotium is a hardened mass of compact mycelial tissue. As is common practice in TCM, the mushrooms or sclerotia were decocted, usually as part of a formulation. A decoction, or tea, has the benefit of being concentrated and fast-acting. In the case of these fungi, decoctions also break down cell walls, allowing the medicinal components to become available and thereby readily absorbed once consumed.

Laboratory analysis indicates that *Poria cocos* has anti-leukemia activity and it may have anti-tumor potential as well. An extract of the sclerotium of *Poria cocos* was as active as etoposide, a major chemotherapeutic drug, in inhibiting a human carcinoma cell line. Another study showed that *Poria cocos* has anti-inflammatory activity that may be useful in inflammatory skin conditions such as psoriasis. *Poria cocos* is shown to have anti-inflammatory activity when taken orally or applied topically. Recently, two patents have been approved for the use of *Poria cocos* in skin creams for the treatment of oily skin and acne and for sun-damaged skin. The women of the Imperial Chinese court used *Poria cocos* in skin treatments to moisturize, nourish, help prevent pimples, and to promote "radiant" skin. It is also thought to help prevent dark spots and wrinkles.

Poria cocos is the main component of many Chinese medicinal combination drugs that have therapeutic effects on recurrent spontaneous abortion and that can help maintain pregnancy until delivery. It was hypothesized that this herbal medicine can also prolong organ survival after transplantation. A group from Harbin, China, recently reported on the anti-rejection effect of the extract of *Poria cocos* in rats after cardiac allograft implantation. Acute rejection of heart transplants and cellular immune reaction can be effectively suppressed using this extract of *Poria cocos*.

ROZITES CAPERATA

Rozites caperata is a delicious edible mushroom known as the gypsy. *Rozites* is named in honor of a European mycologist Ernst Roze, who worked in the early 1900s. The specific epithet *caperata* means wrinkled—older specimens of this mushroom often have a wrinkled cap. This mushroom grows in northern zones throughout the world, especially with conifers, but sometimes in mixed hardwoods such as oak, birch, and aspen. It is a popular and delicious edible mushroom, but it should not be collected by beginners, since it could easily be confused with several poisonous mushrooms.

Frank Piraino, a retired virologist from the University of Wisconsin-Madison and avid mushroom hobbyist, initially noted the antiviral activity of this mushroom more than 40 years ago. Piraino tested the *Rozites caperata* extract on a strain of chicken leukemia, the only virus at his disposal while working with the Milwaukee Health Department in 1964. Cultures treated with the mushroom extract did not develop tumors. When Piraino joined St. Joseph's Hospital in the 1980s, he was able to continue screening the mushroom with additional viruses, showing that *Rozites caperata* was effective against influenza A, chicken pox, herpes simplex virus types 1 and 2, and respiratory syncytial virus (RSV). He has since isolated an active ingredient in the mushroom; the antiviral effects cannot be obtained by simply eating *Rozites caperata*.

TREMELLA FUCIFORMIS

Snow fungus (*Tremella fuciformis*; also known as white fungus, snow fungus, or silver tree-ear fungus) is a type of jelly fungus (a kind of mushroom) that is used in Chinese cuisine. In Chinese, it is called *yin er* ("silver ear") or *bai mu er* ("white wood ear"), and in Japanese it is called *shiro kikurage* ("white tree jellyfish"). The fungus grows in frilly masses on trees and is off-white in color and very translucent.

Wild versions of the fungus are rather small, about the size of a golf ball. Since it was found growing on wood in nature, it was assumed that this fungus was using the wood for its nutrition. Eventually, studies in fungal ecology revealed that *Tremella* species are mycoparasites—they don't eat the wood but rather another fungus that is eating the wood. In this case, the host fungus is *Hypoxylon archeri*, one of the black Pyrenomycetes, all of which are wood decay fungi.

The mushroom product is often purchased dried and must be soaked before usage. It is used in both savory and sweet dishes. While tasteless, it is enjoyed for its jelly-like texture as well as its purported medicinal benefits. It can be sautéed in olive oil and butter (after rehydration), until browned and just a bit crispy, and it can even be prepared as a dessert.

The snow fungus has been eaten for centuries in China, where it is considered to have significant medicinal properties, having been used against tuberculosis, high blood pressure, and even the common cold. Researchers have attributed the medicinal effects of *Tremella* to the polysaccharide content of the mushrooms, especially acidic glucuronoxylomannans. There seems to be some antitumor properties attributable to the stimulation of the immune system by these polysaccharides. *Tremella* species also seem to possess antidiabetic, anti-inflammatory, and antiallergic activities, lowers cholesterol, and protects the liver. *Tremella* glucuronoxylomannan may also improve immunodeficiency, including that induced by AIDS, stress, or aging. And it may help maintain better blood flow to vital organs with aging.

Glucuronoxylomannan from the fruiting bodies of *Tremella fuciformis* exhibited a significant dose-dependent hypoglycemic effect in normal mice and also showed a significant activity in diabetic mice. It reduced the glycogen content in the liver, increased the total lipid in adipose tissue, and lowered the plasma cholesterol level. The hypoglycemic activity of *Tremella fuciformis* in normal mice was responsible for an increase of insulin secretion and for the acceleration of glucose metabolism. Continuous oral administration was found to be the most effective route for both normal and diabetic mice.

Three heteroglycans, T1a, T1b, and T1c, have been isolated from the body of *Tremella fuciformis*. They have been shown to induce human white blood cells to produce interleukin-1 (IL-1), interleukin-6 (IL-6), and tumor necrosis factor (TNF), a significant immunostimulating potential. Most of these effects come from long-term consumption of the fungus.

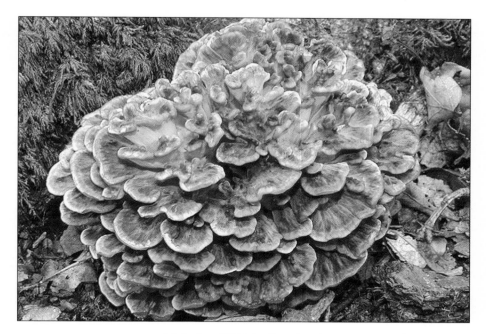

Maitake *(Grifola frondosa)*

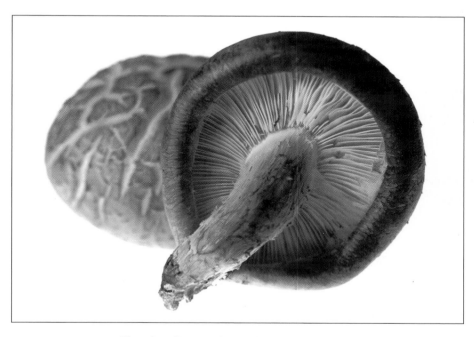

Shitake *(Lentinula* or *Lentinus edodes)*

PLATE 1

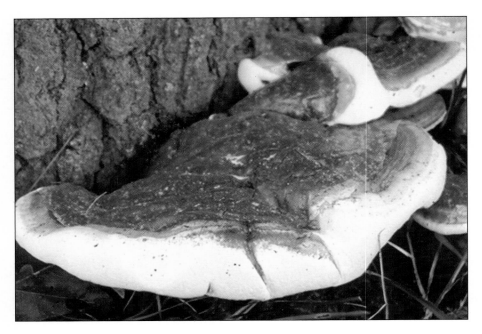

Reishi *(Ganoderma lucidum)*

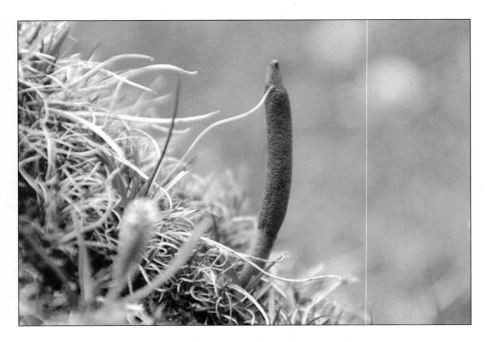

Cordyceps sinensis

PLATE 2

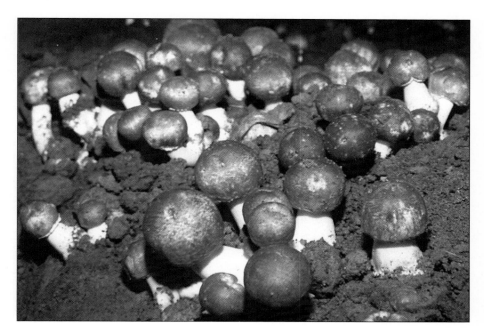

Agaricus blazei

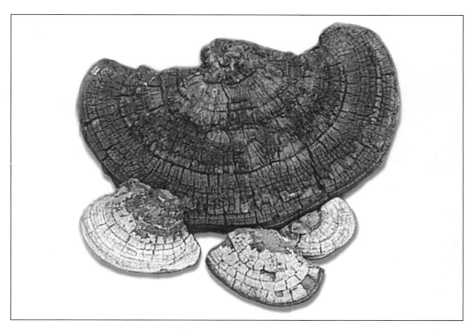

Phellinus linteus

PLATE 3

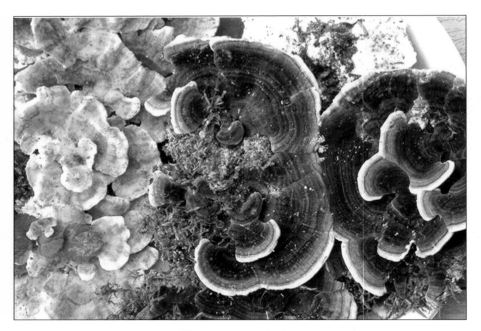

Trametes versicolor

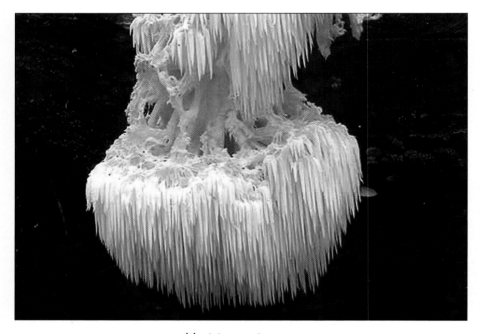

Hericium erinaceus

PLATE 4

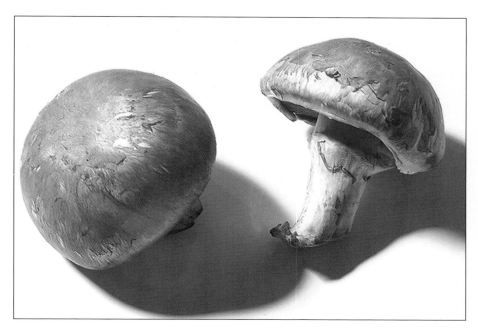

Agaricus bisporus

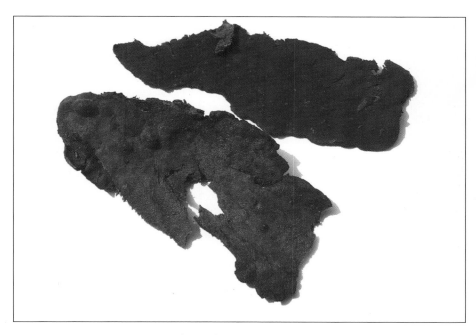

Antrodia camphorata

PLATE 5

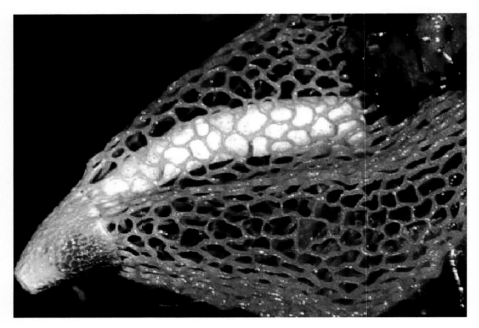

Dictyophora indusiata

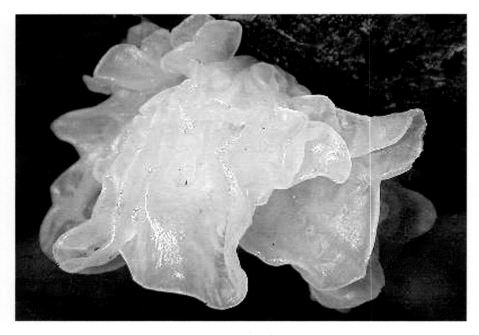

Tremella fuciformis

PLATE 6

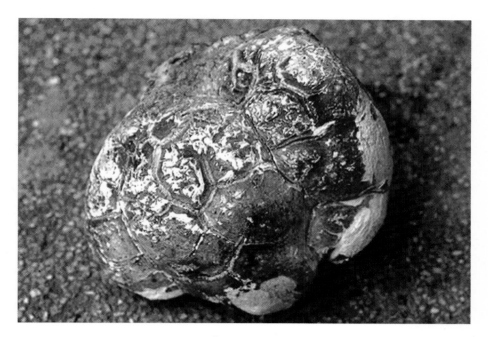

Poria cocos

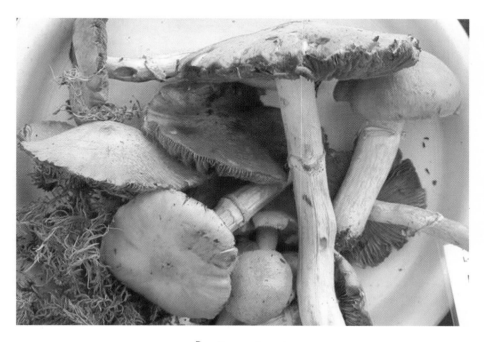

Rozites caperata

PLATE 7

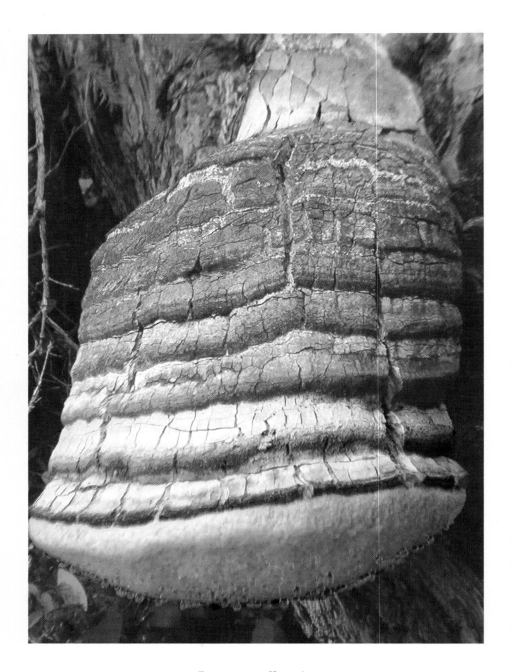

Fomitopis officinalis

PLATE 8

13

Mushroom Cultivation

For many centuries, foraging for and picking mushrooms in the wild was the only way to obtain them. Sometime in the first millennium, however, cultivators in Japan and China began using the log method to grow mushrooms. With this technique, logs from felled trees are placed next to a stump or log where the fruit-bodies of mushrooms grow. The idea is for spores from the fruit-body to find their way to the felled trees and spawn a new crop. The log method is still practiced in parts of China. People use it to supplement their incomes and produce mushrooms for local markets.

More controlled methods of cultivation begin in the 1930s. At that time, Japanese cultivators began growing mushrooms on logs wrapped in rice straw. The farmer would find a log with reishi or shiitake growing on it, cut a slice from the log, and sandwich the log between other logs. Then the farmer would bind all the logs in rice straw. Soon the spores from the infected log would infect the other logs as well and mushrooms would begin growing on all the logs.

The log method of cultivating mushrooms worked very well, but then farmers hit on the idea of burying an infected log in the soil. With this technique, the log retained moisture longer, which encouraged the mushrooms to grow. What's more, the log wasn't exposed to and infected by unwanted weed fungi. Another cultivation method is to place mycelium from a mushroom on a wooden plug, drill a small hole in a log, hammer the plug into the log, and wax over the small hole to keep foreign spores out.

Recently, with the popularity of mushrooms on the rise and demand for mushrooms at an all-time high, cultivators have sought more advanced techniques for controlled cultivation. One technique is to cultivate the mushrooms in sawdust. This way, the fruit-bodies of the shiitake mushroom, for example, grow in 90 days, whereas cultivating the mushroom on logs requires 18 months.

Another technique is to cultivate the mushrooms on grains such as brown rice, barley, or buckwheat. The grains are sterilized and placed into special bags or jars that allow the mycelium to breathe but keep contaminants out. The pristine environment is essential. By the end of the growth cycle, the mycelium has eaten the grain and digested it. As long as the grower's technique is good, very little of the grain remains intact.

In Asia, where demand for medicinal mushroom products is especially high and the products are produced en masse, growers have been devising state-of-the-art techniques to cultivate mycelium. One technique is to grow the mycelium in a liquid culture. Mushroom cultures are introduced into a liquid broth. The growers are quite secretive about their techniques, but suffice it to say, the culture is harvested from the liquid medium and dried into a powder.

Mycologists and growers often tout the superior qualities of the strains they produce. A mushroom strain is a culture from a particular mushroom. Mycologists obtain mushroom strains in various ways. The majority purchase them from a mycological culture bank such as the one run by American Type Culture Collection, a company that provides biological products to science and industry. Mycologists often trade cultures among themselves, and many have large collections in libraries.

Diligent and meticulous mycologists, however, prefer to obtain the strains from mushrooms they collect themselves in the wild. These mycologists, who strive for the highest-quality mushroom, believe that seeing a mushroom in its native environment and acquainting yourself with its special features is essential. Where a mushroom grows, how quickly it grows, and its virulency matter.

CULTIVATION AND THE SAFETY OF MEDICINAL MUSHROOMS

The safety of mushroom-based dietary supplements is enhanced because of the following considerations:

- The overwhelming majority of mushrooms used as dietary supplements are cultivated commercially and not gathered in the wild. This guarantees proper identification, and probably unadulterated products. In many cases, it also means one simple strain. This may also benefit conservation of biodiversity.

- Mushrooms are easily propagated vegetatively, and thus keep to one clone. The mycelium can be stored for a long time, and the biochemical and genetic consistency can be checked after a long period of time.

- Many medicinal and edible mushrooms can be grown as mycelial biomass in submerged cultures, as done in Asia.

- Many growers are experimenting with substrates that have added functional benefits for the final raw material, such as high-antioxidant purple corn or barley with high beta-glucan levels. These increase the amounts of active mushroom components and add their own health-promoting benefits. This process offers organic certification for the raw material, something that the proponents of submerged fermentation have not yet achieved.

This last aspect offers a promising future for standardized production of safe mushroom-based dietary supplements. Submerged culture and semi-solid state fermentation have more consistent and predictable composition than that of fruit bodies. For most substances, this mycelium biomass obtained by submerged cultivation also has higher nutritional value. The culture media in which mycelium grows are made of chemically pure and ecologically clean substances. The cultivation of mushrooms for fruit-body production is a long-term process, taking one to several months for the first fruiting bodies to appear, depending on species and substrate. By contrast, the growth of pure mushroom cultures in submerged conditions in a liquid culture medium permits acceleration of the growth speed, resulting in biomass yield in several days. The additional advantage of submerged culturing is the fact that many medicinal mushrooms do not produce fruiting bodies under commercial cultivation.

Reliable industrial cultivation techniques are known for only 37 mushroom species, but medicinal mushrooms include many species that need several years for development of normal fruiting bodies on trees. Such species cannot be grown commercially, but their mycelia can be grown easily and economically with the help of submerged culturing. High stability and standardization of mycelium grown in submerged cultures is important not only for producing dietary supplements, but also might be beneficial for producing mushroom-based medicines.

The use of medicinal mushrooms goes hand in hand with development of their artificial cultivation. The most significant aspect of mushroom cultivation, if managed properly, is to create zero emissions (no waste). Since more than 70% of agricultural and forest materials are non-productive and are wasted in processing, this is a very real advantage. Many of these waste materials can be used as substrates to grow mushrooms and protect the environment.

EXPERIMENTAL CULTIVATION METHODS

Mushroom cultivation has reached new heights of sophistication in recent years, with producers going to great lengths to replicate the growing environment of mushrooms in the laboratory. For example, the *Cordyceps* species is found in oxygen-deficient environments. *Cordyceps* grows in the Himalayas, in swampy areas where high levels of methane and carbon dioxide are found, and in valleys around volcanoes. Because *Cordyceps* grows in these oxygen-deficient environments, it must use oxygen in a very efficient manner. Mycologists experimenting with *Cordyceps* in their laboratories discovered that they could produce higher quantities of Cordycepin by depriving *Cordyceps* mycelium of a certain amount of oxygen. Cordycepin is used to treat bacterial infections such as tuberculosis and leprosy as well as inhibiting HIV replication.

The mushroom-growing industry has devoted itself to producing larger fruit-bodies and consistent crops of mushroom fruit-bodies. Not many producers have turned their attention to producing chemical compounds from mushrooms. When mycologists experiment with producing compounds in their mushrooms, they change the growth parameters and get some odd-looking fruit-bodies. These mushrooms would not be marketable in the culinary market as shiitakes, for instance, because they're ugly and pink. But these mycologists are trying to produce Lentinan, Krestin, Cordycepin, and other compounds more efficiently.

Mycologists can use advanced techniques in analytical chemistry to quickly, accurately, and relatively inexpensively test the compounds in mushrooms. They can find out what these compounds are with a degree of certainty never known before. For that matter, they can discover new compounds. The new technologies will be especially useful in the emerging field of mapping beta-glucan structures. What was assumed in the past can actually be quantified. We can expect to discover new compounds, some of which will serve to prevent or cure disease, in the years ahead.

CULTIVATING MYCELIUM IN THE LABORATORY

Using cell-culture technology, it is now possible to grow mushroom mycelium (the feeding body of the mushroom that grows beneath the soil) in the laboratory. The processes for growing mycelium are very technical, but suffice it to say that the mycelium is produced in much the same way that baker's and brewer's yeasts are produced. Given the right environment and conditions, mycelium made in the laboratory has the same biological activity as mycelium that is grown in the wild. What's more, it is cleaner and more potent.

Recently, scientists Randy Dorian of Hanuman Medical, in San Francisco, and Moshe Shifrine, of Santa Fe, New Mexico, succeeded in cultivating truffles (*Tuber melanosporum*) in liquid culture. The scientists used mammalian cell tissue culturing techniques to grow fungal tissue. Their success was verified through DNA analysis. Truffles contain many interesting compounds that may have significant value as nutraceuticals.

From the health-conscious consumer's point of view, maybe the best thing about laboratory-produced mycelium is its cost. *Cordyceps* mushrooms, for example, cost as much as $10,000 per kilogram. By contrast, most pharmacies and health food stores sell a *Cordyceps* powder that is significantly less expensive than that, making mushrooms and mushroom products affordable for everyone.

14

A Buyer's Guide to Mushrooms

I t has been estimated that worldwide sales of dietary supplements from medicinal mushrooms are over $7 billion per year; shiitake and reishi sell the most. However, there is currently no standard protocol for guaranteeing medicinal mushroom supplements quality and efficacy. Medicinal mushrooms have been used for centuries or, in some cases, for thousands of years. There are few documented adverse effects to man and as such they can be considered as safe. Any compound that will influence body functions, such as blood pressure, immune response, and so on, is classified as a pharmacological agent, and as such will invariably demonstrate toxicity at high dosage levels. Thus, a completely safe pharmacological agent would not have any biological activity. However, from a pharmacological point of view, safety is a relative concept and it is clear that the safety of all mushroom-derived dietary supplements cannot be guaranteed simply because they have many centuries of usage.

VARIABLE QUALITY

Anyone who shops for mushrooms or mushroom products must be aware that some products are better than others. The last decade or so has seen a large increase in the number of mushroom farms, especially in the northwestern United States, where the climate is damp and conducive to growing mushrooms. On some occasions, the people who manage these farms, while well intentioned, produce mushrooms of inferior quality because they start from weak isolates. The problem is that most of the mushrooms are grown from hybridized strains and these strains have only a five-year to eight-year life span. After that, they weaken and their bioefficiency drops.

The grower gets the mushroom strain from a supplier and reproduces it. At first, the growing is successful, but the success rate will decline unless the grower knows how to maintain the strain under laboratory conditions. That is a delicate matter requiring more expertise than most people have. We have observed that books about cultivating mushrooms usually offer advice for growing or harvesting, but offer little in the way of how to maintain the original fungus, and that is the crucial issue. In the future, we hope that organizations that present mushroom-growing seminars to amateur mycologists will include in-depth training in long-term culture maintenance.

Because temperature and climate are so important in mushroom cultivation, Japanese suppliers have been creating strains especially for use in different climates. In Kyushu Province, where it is warmer, one strain is used; in the northern, colder part of the country, growers use a different strain. Different strains for different climates is nothing new in the world of agriculture. After all, strains of apple, cherry, and all other fruit trees are planted where they will grow best. However, many American mushroom growers are not as sophisticated as they could be and are not taking climate into account.

Another thing for consumers of mushroom products to consider is how the mycelium is handled. The mycelium is the feeding body of the mushroom that grows underground. Preferably, mushroom mycelium should be processed from start to finish on the same site. Mushroom mycelium is a fragile substance. When it is jostled about or moved from place to place, it can be shocked and bruised, which inhibits its healthy growth cycle. The ideal mycelium mushroom product is harvested at the peak of its vigor and processed immediately on site.

Mushrooms are great absorbers. Like sponges, they take in what is in their environment. Growers who adhere to organic growing procedures produce mushrooms of the highest purity. For that reason, mushroom products that originate in the United States are preferable to mushroom products that originate in industrialized areas in other parts of the world, where pollution and environmental toxins are often more prevalent.

MULTIPLE-MUSHROOM SUPPLEMENTS

Anyone who goes to the health food store in search of mushroom products inevitably finds what the health food industry calls "multiple-mushroom formulas." Each formula is a mixture of three to as many as 14 different

Mushrooms in the Mainstream

Recently, bakers in the San Francisco Bay Area have begun experimenting with the use of medicinal mushroom mycelium cultivated on whole grains. The mycelium powder can be blended in flour and used in baking. As the whole-grain mycelium is heated during the baking process, its beta-glucans become more bioavailable. In other words, they are made easier to digest. Putting whole-grain mushroom mycelium in baked goods is a novel and effective way to take the mushrooms, especially where children are concerned, since young-sters often balk at taking pills and capsules. On many occasions, we have put reishi and *Agaricus blazei* mycelium powder in our families' pancake mix with-out anyone being the wiser.

Contemporary cuisine has begun to make use of culinary mushrooms. Oys-ter mushrooms (*Pleurotus ostreatus*), maitakes, Pom Pom Blancs (*Hericium erinaceus*), and *Agaricus blazei* are now showing up in the kitchens of some of America's best chefs. Apart from their medicinal value, these mushrooms are delicious. They are often the defining element in the dish in which they are served. Savvy chefs are proudly pointing out to their clientele that they are get-ting something rare and valuable—a food that has been revered since ancient times for its flavor as well as its health-giving properties.

Now that the general public in the United States and other formerly myco-phobic countries are beginning to embrace mushrooms, we hope to see more mushrooms in the diet and more mushroom additives in food. Recently, a fun-gus-based meat substitute marketed under the brand name Quorn has appeared on the shelves of some markets. Quorn has been popular in Europe for some time and recently received Food and Drug Administration approval in the Unit-ed States. The product, made from the fungus *Fusarium venenatum,* is sup-posed to taste, of course, like chicken.

mushrooms in powder form. The idea is to cover as many bases as possi-ble in a single formula. Reishi, shiitake, *Cordyceps*, and other medicinal mushrooms each offer different health benefits. The different polysaccha-ride structures, terpenoids, and other unique active substances in the dif-ferent mushrooms trigger unique receptors of the immune system, or target receptors on microbes or malignant cells. The idea is to feed the body a lot of different active substances derived from unique mushroom sources to lift the immune system relatively quickly.

Each mushroom appears to produce its own unique type of beta-glucan and terpenoids. One may stimulate the production of T cells while another helps natural killer cells do their job. *Agaricus blazei,* for example, stimulates the production of natural killer cells. Maitake stimulates the production of T cells. By putting both mushrooms in the mix, you stimulate T cells and natural killer cells.

If you prefer to take a multiple-mushroom formula, read the label to find out how much of each mushroom is in the formula. Also, note what percentage of the formula is composed of each mushroom. Incidences of bad reactions to a medicinal mushroom are very rare. Usually, when someone has a bad reaction, the cause is a lack of an enzyme for digesting a particular mushroom. Very few anaphylactic reactions have ever been recorded when taking medicinal mushrooms. For these reasons, mixing many kinds of mushrooms into a formula is safe.

But even multiple-mushroom formulas may not be enough. Recent research has demonstrated that a synergistic effect—the combination will be more effective than the sum of the parts—has been consistently observed when subjects with high blood sugar or high blood pressure were taking a multiple-mushroom formula with other well-documented active natural substances. For example, in high blood sugar, the addition of the Indian plant *Salacia oblonga,* cinnamon, biotin, and chromium to a mushroom formula has resulted in more constantly reliable clinical results.

Research on Multiple-Mushroom Formulas

Researchers in the United States along with Chinese scientists conducted a clinical trial with a multiple-mushroom formula in the People's Hospital of Lishui City, in Zhejiang Province, China. The formula consisted of powder in tablet form from six mushrooms: *Agaricus blazei,* shiitake, maitake, reishi, *Trametes versicolor,* and *Cordyceps sinensis.* The study was conducted on 56 patients in the middle to late stages (Stage 3 and 4) of cancer. In terms of their physical condition, white blood cell count, granular leukocyte count, and appetite, the subjects of the study were similar. Thirty patients were given 6 grams per day of the multiple-mushroom formula and 26 patients were given 30 milligrams a day of the drug Polyactin-A.

Rather than give the comparison group a placebo, as is the custom in the West, Chinese physicians prefer to give the comparison group a medicine. Although this makes the results of experiment harder to assess, Chinese physicians believe for ethical reasons that giving comparison groups some kind of treatment is necessary. All patients in the study were treated concurrently with radiotherapy or chemotherapy a week after they began taking either the multiple-mushroom formula or Polyactin-A. Both groups took their medications for a total of two months.

At the end of the trial period, the multiple-mushroom group showed improvements beyond those of the comparison group. The scientists wrote that the mixed mushroom polysaccharides "can inhibit the protein synthesis of cancer cells, change the physiological condition of cancer cells, inhibit the growth and transference of cancer cells, relieve the poisoning action of anticancer drugs, improve the patients' sleep and appetite, and result in overall improvement of the symptoms." The scientists concluded that the curative effect of the multiple-mushroom formula was higher than that of Polyactin-A and that it can serve a helper role in the treatment of tumor patients.

Multiple Mushrooms and High Blood Pressure

As we grow older, we are more likely to suffer from high blood pressure (hypertension). The disorder is caused by tension, or pressure, on the arteries that constricts the flow of blood and makes the heart work harder. The causes of hypertension are hard to pinpoint. Most people inherit the disorder from their parents. Corpulence, poor diet, lack of exercise, stress, and environmental factors can also play a role. Interestingly, the disorder is much more prevalent in industrialized societies than underdeveloped ones.

Researchers at Tohoku University, in Japan, experimented with hypertensive rats to gauge the effect of maitake and shiitake mushrooms on blood pressure. For eight weeks, one group was fed maitake along with its normal diet, another group was fed shiitake, and a third group received no mushroom supplement. After eight weeks, when the groups were compared, researchers discovered that blood pressure in the maitake-fed group had lowered. However, there was no difference between the maitake and control groups in terms of cholesterol levels, triglyceride levels, or plasma levels. By contrast, blood pressure readings were not lower in the shiitake-fed group; however, levels of plasma and triglyceride were lower.

This experiment demonstrates the value of multiple-mushroom formulas. And the combination of maitake, reishi, and Cordyceps may be more regularly active than each mushroom extract individually. Here, you can see the benefits of taking more than one mushroom to receive the medicinal effects of different mushrooms.

EXTRACT, CAPSULE, OR POWDER?

Essentially there are three ways to take medicinal mushroom products: as an extract, capsule, or powder. Medicinal mushrooms in capsule form come from dried and powdered mycelium. The mycelium is ground into a powder and encapsulated or pressed into pills. In extract form, water and alcohol are used to extract the active constituents of the mycelium. Water, for instance, extracts beta-glucans. In the case of reishi, alcohol is used to extract the triterpenes, the elements that aid the cardiovascular system. The extract is then bottled and sold in health food stores.

Whether you take a mushroom product in extract, capsule, or powder

---

Tips on Buying Mushroom Supplements

When selecting among commercially available mushroom extracts and supplements, look for and be careful about the following factors.

• Safety: Make sure that the product you buy is free of toxic contaminants, such as heavy metals (lead, cadmium, mercury, arsenic). Look for a U.S. Department of Agriculture (USDA)–certified organic product. Also, the state of California has its own, very strict certification program, and some products may have kosher certification.

• Consistency and Quality Control: The manufacturer should be able to provide evidence of regular, independent laboratory evaluation showing that from batch to batch you are getting the same active product. Quality control is expensive, but it is your best guarantee for safety and effectiveness. Make sure that the manufacturer complies with U.S. Food and Drug Administration (FDA) Good Manufacturing Practices (GMPs).

• Form: There are many supplement forms available—drops, liquid extracts with or without alcohol, powder in capsules, softgels, and lacquered tablets. Choose the form that you like best!

• Combinations and Multiple Mushroom Formulas: Combination formulas are becoming more popular. One reason is that multiple mushroom formulas, and combinations with other natural substances, help to restore balance instead of attacking a symptom. Balance or harmony is a central benefit that you can expect from mushrooms. A good combination, even a small amount, will pack more benefits than a number of separate large capsules—an illustration of the notion of synergy.

form doesn't matter in terms of the health benefits. What matters is which form you are most comfortable taking. Some companies believe that fermentation of medicinal mushrooms with probiotic cultures—yogurt cultures such as *Lactobacillus acidophilus* and *Bacillus bifidus*—make the mushrooms easier to digest, especially for people whose digestive systems are impaired.

In the United States, most manufacturers use cheap gelatin or vegetable capsules—you can open these and mix the powder with food or liquid. But these capsules are sensitive to humidity and heat: in an area where temperatures may rise above 100°F or humidity is high, the capsule and its contents will suffer, unless they are individually blister-packed with additional Aclar® Film protection for optimum moisture barrier and stability. That's why some manufacturers are using "softgel" capsules, which can encapsulate liquid extracts, are highly resistant to temperature and humidity variations, and are easy to swallow. A number of companies now use softgels for mushroom and other natural extracts.

Recent improvements in pharmaceutical technology has resulted in the advent of lacquered tablets. These tablets can be programmed to release the active ingredients they contain either rapidly (peak blood levels), slowly (achieving steady serum concentration), or in any other desired timed-release fashion. They are highly resistant to changes in temperature or humidity and have a shelf-life exceeding five years. They can also contain nanoparticles for even better systemic delivery. Some manufacturers are now offering these nanotechnology-improved lacquered tablets for medicinal mushroom extracts, such as Swisscaps, headquartered in Kirchberg, Switzerland.

A FINAL WORD ABOUT PRICES AND SAFETY

As a raw material, medicinal mushrooms are more expensive than most of the other herbal supplements that you can buy in health food stores. The price of a quality medicinal mushroom product runs between $12 and $100 for a one-month supply, depending on the quality and number of strains in the formula. If you encounter a mushroom product that costs less than $10, you should be wary. As they become popular, more and more mushroom products are appearing on the market, and some of these products are of inferior quality. Before you purchase a medicinal mushroom product, do your homework and find the one from which you will obtain the most health benefits. However, that product will probably cost more.

Another caveat is the quality of the mushroom extract. As you already know, mushrooms are scavengers: they collect and neutralize (for themselves only) toxins, toxic heavy metals, and other by-products. Therefore, it is very important with mushroom extracts (possibly more than with any other supplement) to be sure of purity and cleanliness. I strongly advise you to look for U.S. Department of Agriculture (USDA) organic certification. This may make the difference between safety and toxicity, not to mention guaranteed efficacy. The USDA organic certification must be printed on the supplement box and on the container itself.

Conclusion

Ever since my father taught me about *cèpes,* chanterelles, and other mushrooms as a boy, I have been fascinated by these odd and often delicious fungi. While in refugee camps in Switzerland during World War II, I remember hoping for rain during the late summer or early fall, so I could visit the hidden places where mushrooms would sprout. I will always recall the secret joy of those occasions with fondness. Many of you were no doubt similarly entranced as children at the sudden, magical appearance of mushrooms after a summer rain.

Fungi are essential for a healthy forest: if there are no fungi in the soil, plants cannot grow, because they cannot break down and absorb nutrients without the help of fungi. Mushrooms have also proven essential for human health. They have been used as medicines by humans around the globe for over 5,000 years. And this book has shown you why they are a perennial favorite on the dinner table and in the medicine cabinet. Modern science is now confirming that mushrooms contain a large array of nutrients and other natural ingredients that boost the immune system, fight infections, and have anti-cancer properties. They help control blood pressure, balance glucose levels and lipids in the blood, promote healthy teeth and gums, optimize liver function, control appetite and weight, boost sex drive and fertility, and much more.

There are over 1,500,000 species of fungi on earth and mushrooms constitute perhaps as many as 22,000 known species. But this may be less than 10% of the total. There may be thousands of as yet undiscovered species that will be of possible benefit to humankind. Even among the known species the number of well-investigated mushrooms is very low. If medicinal mushrooms have a very long tradition to build on, they are also the potential source of exciting and promising treatments in the future.

In the distant human past, all plants and animals were seen as repositories of secret power that could be used for good or ill. In a sense, the whole world was a pharmacopoeia. Mushrooms have always been part of this legendary past. Now, we can look forward to new discoveries in the years to come, when modern science will harness the medicinal powers of mushrooms for the good of us all.

It is my sincerest hope that you will use the information in this book to improve your own health. However, this book is just a first step in your request for best health. Use the knowledge you have gained from reading these pages to take the next step. I encourage you to visit shops or recommended Websites that carry these mushrooms and their related products. Use them to see for yourself whether you can benefit from them directly. The more options you have to choose from, the more likely you will be to find what you are looking for. And on top of it all, many mushrooms are delicious! Humankind has been nourished by medicinal mushrooms for many centuries. And since many mushrooms are delicacies while also delivering better health, enjoy them!

Bon Appétit et Bonne Santé.

Resources

For readers interested in incorporating mushrooms into their diet or supplement program, here is a select list of mushroom resources. Fresh mushrooms, of course, are available in most grocery stores, with higher-end natural food stores having more varieties. You can add mushrooms to stir-fries, meat dishes, salads, and many other prepared foods in order to incorporate their healing benefits into your diet. Mushroom supplements can be found in grocery stores, in health food stores, over the Internet, and even in drug stores. For those interested in mushroom hunting, most bookstores carry field guides (a short list appears on page 140) or you might consider joining your local mycological society and taking a class to learn more. Consult the organizations listed below or check www.mykoweb.com/na_mycos.html for a list of local mycological societies.

As mentioned in many chapters of this book, buying commercially available medicinal mushrooms extracts can be tricky. Let me remind you what you must look for, and be careful about:

Safety: Make sure that the product you buy is free of toxic contaminants, like heavy metals (lead, cadmium, mercury, arsenic). Best is to look for a USDA-certified organic product. The state of California has its own, very strict, certification. Some products also have Kosher certification, but all mushrooms are, by definition, kosher, unless they are grown on pork or horse meat, or in mollusk farms!

Consistency: The manufacturer should be able to provide evidence of regular, independent laboratory evaluation, showing that from batch to batch, from January 1st until December 31st, you are getting the same identical, active product.

Quality Control: QC—as we call it—is expensive, but it is your best guarantee. Make sure that the factory or the plant complies with Good Manufacturing Practices (GMPs). For mushroom extracts, GMPs are "Food," not "Pharmaceuticals," but they are strict. In some countries, e.g. Taiwan, Korea or China, medicinal mushroom extract currently manufactured must comply with Pharmaceutical GMPs.

Presentation: There are many presentations available: drops or liquid extracts (by the teaspoon), with or without alcohol; capsules that contain a powder that can be mixed with a beverage or food; softgels; and lacquered tablets that are very popular because of their long shelf life and ease for swallowing. Choose the presentation that you like best!

Nanotechnology: Nanoparticles are very, very tiny: a nanometer is one billionth of a meter (one meter is just a bit longer than a yard). These particles are very tiny indeed, and can be absorbed much better than just ground mushrooms; they can even enter cells and their nuclei. Modern nanotechnology has recently focused on natural substances, and the Department of Applied Biology and Chemical Technology at the Hong Kong Polytechnic University has developed such extracts.

Combinations, Multiple Mushroom formulas, & Synergy:

These are becoming more popular by the day. One reason is that multiple mushrooms combinations, along with other natural substances, help to restore balance instead of attacking a symptom or even a disease. The concept of "balance" or "harmony" is central to the effects and benefits that you can expect from mushrooms. Fairly often, a tradition-based formula, using USDA-certified organic products and packaged under the strictest conditions of cleanliness and modern delivery system, will help you, while a lower quality product will only result in disagreeable side effects.

Synergy was explained in Chapter 4. As you read, sometimes a small volume of an adequate combination of mushrooms will pack more benefits than a number of separate large capsules—even absorbed within minutes. This is the magic of modern science and technology!

But where can you order the best mushroom extracts, multiple formulas, and synergistic combinations? If you search the Internet, you will find hundreds of websites that look very attractive. Each will use seductive language to get your business. I have made a very limited selection of companies that you can trust. I have omitted many that are certainly excellent, but these could not display the comprehensive information that you deserve. I have not included any information on growing your own mushrooms: you will never recoup your investment—and there are already so many excellent suppliers!

Hereunder are the companies you can trust, in alphabetical order.

NORTH AMERICA

Sources for Mushrooms and Mushroom Supplements

Aloha Medicinals, Inc.

This is America's largest producer of organic medicinal mushrooms. Aloha Medicinals is the actual manufacturer of its products, and manufactures for many other compa-

nies (so-called "private labels"). All its products are fully USDA Certified Organic. It uses only organically grown (certified organic by third-party group California Certified Organic Farmers), non-irradiated, non-GMO mushrooms and plants. It uses no fillers, preservatives or additives in its products. Recently, Aloha Medicinals has been selected to be the exclusive distributor of "Pure and Clean of Switzerland," a line of unique products described on the website www.pureandcleanofswitzerland.com. These products combine the traditional wisdom of China, the USDA certified organic quality, and the strictest controlled modern technology of Switzerland.
P.O. Box 686, Haiku, HI 96708
Phone: 877-508-1077 (orders)

Research and Manufacturing Facility:
1211 Fair Avenue, Santa Cruz, CA 95060
Phone: 831-426-2059

African Division:
Aloha Medicinals (GH) Ltd.
P.O. Box AH 257 Achimota, Accra, Ghana, West Africa
Website: www.alohamedicinals.com
Customer Service E-mail: info@alohamedicinals.com
Technical and Research E-mail: research@alohamedicinals.com

Birkdale Medicinals, Inc.
The US source for the product that is being used throughout Africa as a medicine for the treatment of HIV and AIDS. Named Immune Assist 247, this is not an FDA-approved drug in America, but is an all-natural, USDA Certified Organic non-toxic supplement that may help many patients manage their disease for the long term. Birkdale also distributes other U.S.-manufactured quality Medicinal Mushroom formulations for use as daily supplements.
250 North Newman Road, Lake Orion, MI 48362
Phone: 248-693-8211
Website: www.immuneassist247.com

Functional Fungi LLC.
One of the leaders in medicinal fungi cultivation and innovation. As a California-based raw material supplier for manufacturers in the dietary supplement and nutraceutical industries, Functional Fungi offers exceptional quality, USDA-certified organic, Kosher-certified medicinal, and completely vegetarian mushroom raw material for the nutraceutical and gourmet foods industries. Functional Fungi currently provides 28 medicinal mushrooms to manufacturers.
P.O. Box 68, Arroyo Grande, CA 93420
Phone: 805-489-4227
Website: www.functionalfungi.com
E-mail: info@functionalfungi.com

Fungi Perfecti® LLC.

A family-owned, environmentally friendly company specializing in gourmet and medicinal mushrooms. Founded by mycologist and author Paul Stamets, Fungi Perfecti is Certified Organic by the Washington State Department of Agriculture. In has been in business since 1980, and offers MycoMedicinals®, mushroom kits, books, and much more.

P.O. Box 7634, Olympia, WA 98507
Phone: 800-780-9126 (orders) or 360-426-9292
Website : www.fungi.com
E-mail: info@fungi.com

Lost Creek Shiitake Mushroom Farm

Shiitake mushroom logs, shiitake soups, dips & gift items.

P.O. Box 520, 9319 South Brush Creek Road, Perkins, OK 74059
Phone: 800-792-0053 (orders) or 405-547-2234
Website: www.shiitakemushroomlog.com
E-mail: ma.and.pa@shiitakemushroomlog.com

Medicinal Mushrooms

Since 1994, provides organic-certified hot water extracts and dried medicinal mushrooms to the industry.

PO Box 50398, Eugene, OR 97405
Phone: 888-283-6583 (orders) or 541-344-8753
Website: http://www.medicinalmushrooms.net/index.html
E-mail: sales@mushroomscience.com

Misty Mountain Specialties

A Canadian company that deals in wild and domestic mushrooms and other specialty forest products.

#108 – 2971 Viking Way, Richmond, BC, V6V 1Y1, Canada
Phone: 604 273-8299
Website: http://www.mistymt.com
E-mail: info@mistymt.com

Mitobi Enterprises Ltd.

Established in 1982, Mitobi sells wholesale large bags of several medicinal mushrooms and even more gourmet ones.

18036 59th Avenue, Surrey, BC V3S 1P7, Canada
Phone: 604 576-8807
Website: http://www.mitobi.com
E-mail: sales@mitobi.com

Modern Mushroom Farms, Inc.

The Ciarrocchi family at Modern Mushroom Farms has been raising mushrooms in Kennett Square, Pennsylvania, the Mushroom Capital of the World, for three

generations. The catalog includes *Agaricus bisporus* as White, Crimini, and Porta-bella; Shiitake, Oyster, Enoki, Maitake and Beech; all are available fresh or dried.
P.O. Box 340, Avondale, PA 19311
Phone: 610-268-3535
Website: www.modernmush.com
E-mail: info@modernmush.com

MycoPharma® from EliteLands

Eight medicinal mushrooms extracts; mycelia are grown on liquid in organic mushroom greenhouses. EliteLands has strict quality controls, and GMP-certified pharmaceutical grade extraction.
2416 NE 88th Avenue, Portland, OR 97220
Phone: 503-860-4740
Website: www.elitelands.com

NAMMEX

Primary supplier of mushroom extracts to the nutritional supplement industry. These extracts are certified organic by Quality Assurance International, QAI, of San Diego, California. Most are imported from China as raw material.
Box 1780, Gibsons, BC, Canada, V0N 1V0
Phone: 604-886-7799
Website: www.nammex.com

Nature's Gift for Life

1303 Summer Terrace Drive, Sugar Land, TX 77479
Phone: 281-937-9002
Website: www.ng4lnutritionals.com
E-mail: sales@ng4lnutritionals.com

Phillips Mushroom Farms

The largest marketer of specialty mushrooms in the U.S., distributing over 35 million pounds of specialty mushrooms annually. In the late 1920s, William W. Phillips pioneered mushroom farming in Kennett Square, PA, "The Mushroom Capital of the World". The Phillips Family, now in its third generation, has been growing top-quality mushrooms ever since. Phillips Mushroom Farms provides fresh mushrooms, as well as many varieties of dried mushrooms.
1011 Kaolin Road, Kenneth Square, PA 1934
Phone:800-722-8818
Website: www.phillipsmushroomfarms.com
E-mail: info@phillipsmushroomfarms.com

Organizations

North American Mycological Association (NAMA)

6615 Tudor Court, Gladstone, OR 97027-1032

Phone: 503-657-7358
Website: www.namyco.org

Mycological Society of America
P.O. Box 7065, Lawrence, KS 66044
Phone: 800-627-0629
Website: www.msafungi.org

Books

Growing Gourmet and Medicinal Mushrooms by Paul Stamets. Berkeley, CA: Ten Speed Press, 2000.

Mushrooms Demystified: A Comprehensive Guide to Fleshy Fungi by David Arora. Berkeley, CA: Ten Speed Press, 1986.

National Audubon Society Field Guide to North American Mushrooms by Gary H. Lincoff. New York: Knopf, 1981.

North American Mushrooms: A Field Guide to Edible and Inedible Fungi by Orson K. Miller Jr. and Hope H. Miller. Guilford, CT: Falcon, 2006.

EUROPE, THE MIDDLE EAST, AND AFRICA

Sources for Mushrooms and Mushroom Supplements

Mushroom Trade (Croatia)
In cooperation with leading exporters & producers, Mushroom Trade can deliver high quality mushrooms from all origins, any type in any form.
Zagreb, Croatia
Phone/Fax +385 1 3631-699
Website: www.mushroosmtrade.com
E-mail: trade@mushroomstrade.com

Walsh Mushrooms (Ireland & England)
Established in 1979, supplying quality mushrooms to the UK market. This service is backed up by its compost business, supplying a base of growers in Ireland and the UK. Harvesting is to individual customer specifications.
Sales and Distribution Division
Vale Park, Evesham, Worc. WR11 6GP, England
Phone: +44 1386 422999
Fax: +44 1386 425279
Website: http://www.walshmushrooms.com
E-mail: info@walshmushrooms.ie

Wozniak Champignons (Poland)
This company has been growing mushrooms since 1982 . Today it is managed by a

young and dynamic team, brother and sister: Anna Woźniak and Andrzej Woźniak.
63-460 Nowe Skalmierzyce, Gniazdów 18, Poland
Phone: +48 503 174 686
Fax: +48 62 762 22 39
Website: http://www.wozniakfood.com.pl/champignons_index.htm
E-mail: office@wozniakfood.com.pl

InnovaMed (Serbia)

Distributes top-quality U.S. manufactured medicinal mushroom supplements throughout the countries of ex-Yugoslavia. All InnovaMed products are USDA-Certified Organic and made in America.
Radojke Lakic #28, Belgrade, Serbia
Phone: ++381-11-2422967
Website: www.my-immunity.com (in Serbo-Croatian)

Pure and Clean of Switzerland SA (Switzerland)

This company aims at the highest standards in the field of medicinal mushroom preparation: GMP High Swiss Standard manufacturer in Switzerland with active ingredients organically grown in the US with USDA certificate. Pure and Clean of Switzerland SA offers 6 different proprietary organic mushroom complex extract with trademark registration, all based on *Cordyceps* and additional active ingredients.
Pure and Clean of Switzerland SA, Via Valegia 44/3, CH-6926 Montagnola, Switzerland
Phone: ++41 91 922-0048
Fax: +41 91 922 02 16
Website: www.pureandcleanofswitzerland.com
E-mail: pure.clean@switzerland.net

Organizations

British Mycological Society
Website: www.britmycolsoc.org.uk

European Mycological Society
Website: www.euromould.org/index.htm

German Society for Medical Mycology
(Deutschsprachige Mykologische Gesellschaft)
Website: www.dmykg.de/start2.html

Mycological Association of Italy
Website: www.micologi.it

Société Mycologique de France
Website: www.mycofrance.org

ASIA

Sources for Mushrooms and Mushroom Supplements

China Monfly Trading Co. Ltd. (China)
A professional exporter of health food additives, dried vegetables, dry pet foods, aquatic feeds and additives, arts & crafts, and other famous local products. Mushroom products include mushroom powder, extracts, polysaccharides from *Ganoderma Lucidum* (Chinese lingzhi, reishi), Agaricus, Shiitake, Maitake, *Coriolus Versicolor*, ground mushroom powder, dried mushrooms, Lingzhi spores powder, capsules, etc.
1-304 JinJia Yuan, No.36 Gong Nong Rd., Cangshan District
Fuzhou, Fujian 350007, China
Phone/Fax: + 86 591-83406639
Website: www.maker88.com
Email: connieloz@163.com

Yuyao Tanifuchang Farm Co., Ltd. (China)
Yuyao Taifuchang Farm Co., Ltd. is a modern hi-tech agriculture enterprise dealing with non-poisonous vegetables, mushrooms and rare medicinal herbs.
Luo Da Ao Village
Ma Zhu Town
YuYao, Zhejiang Province 315450, China
Phone: +86 574 62469850
Fax: +86-574 62460185
Website: http://chinawebs.com/taifuchang/index.htm

Dubai Herbal and Treatment Centre (Dubai, U.A.E.)
Dubai Herbal and Treatment Center in Dubai, United Arab Emirates, is using US manufactured Medicinal Mushroom Supplements in daily practice for the treatment of many serious illnesses.
Dubai Herbal and Treatment Centre
P.O. Box 2666 , Dubai , UAE
Phone: ++971 4 335-1200
Website: www.dubaihtc.com

Chun Jing (Hong Kong) Ltd.
An exclusive distributor in Asia/Far East of all products of Pure and Clean of Switzerland SA. Product of Switzerland, Swiss made.
23/F, 1 Fullerton Centre, 19 Hung To Road, Kwun Tong, Kowloon,
Hong Kong SAR
Phone: +852 2526-4193/ +852 2526-5423
Fax: +852 2304-1111
E-mail: chunjing@chunjing.com.hk
Website: www.chunjing.com.hk

Long Far Herbal Medicine Manufacturing Ltd. (Hong Kong)

Established in 1998, Long Far cooperates with Chinese medicine experts and professional research & developing institutes. It focuses on high quality, pollutant-free, and highest standards. The Long Far group has acquired a GMP standard-compliant pharmaceutical factory and a natural Chinese herbal raw material production base with GAP standards. Long Far also distributes USDA Certified Organic medicinal mushrooms.

14/F, Tower One, Ever Gain Plaza, 88 Container Port Road, Kwai Chung, NT Hong Kong SAR
Phone: ++ 852 3602-2888
Website: www.longfar.com.hk
E-mail: info@longfar.com.hk

Hokuto & MedKinoko Co. (Japan)

E-mail: saiyou@kinoko-hokto.co.jp
Website: www.hokto-kinoko.co.jp

Tai-ai Co., Ltd. (Japan)

Tai-ai has established the mass-cultivation methods of *Agaricus blazei* for the first time on the world. The company has developed and supplied safe functional food products of *Agaricus blazei* one after another.
16-32 Toyama-cho, Niihama, Ehime 702-0823, Japan
Phone: +81 897-43-9000
Fax: +81-897-43-2639
Website: http://www.taiai.co.jp/english.html

Jade International *(Cordyceps sinensis)* (Nepal)

P.O. Box 8975 Epc 4062, Baluwatar, Kathmandu, Bagmati, Nepal

Sang-hwang Health Products *(Phellinus linteus)* (North Korea)

The company can provide *Phellinus linteus* mushrooms (in dried form) to medical institutions, research centers, drug companies and individuals specialized or interested in the treatment of cancer, AIDS, diabetes and other ailments.
Commercial Section
Embassy of the DPR. Korea in Austria, Wien, Austria
Phone: +43 1 523-689622
Fax: +43 1 523-6823
Website: http://www.dprkorea-trade.com/sang/sang01.htm
E-mail: info@dprkorea-trade.com

Lifestream Group Pte. Ltd. (Singapore)

A leading player of functional food and medicinal mushroom products in Singapore and South East Asia, Lifestream Group develops and delivers reliable medicinal mushroom products which are also "100% pure-encapsulated" without additives, fillers and colorant to warrant highest bio-availability and safety for consumers.

GMP certified extraction and manufacturing as well as quality and safety tests from reputable 3rd party laboratories are reasons for its reputation in its market.

Specializing in *Cordyceps,* Lifestream Group, in collaboration with leading U.S. mycologists, developed BRM360°™, a state of the art, proprietary blend of 6 medicinal mushroom extract with Mycoplex-6™, an exclusive blend of full spectrum mushroom compounds, to offer complex heteropolysaccharides compounds for the best therapeutic effects.

KA Place #05-01, 159 Kampong Ampat, Singapore 368328

Phone: + 65 6535-7333

Fax: + 65 6535-7913

Website: http://www.lifestreamgroup.com

E-mail: info@lifestreamgroup.com

MycoBiotech Inc. (Singapore)

Established in 1980 by Dr Kok Kheng Tan, MycoBiotech has pioneered research and development in the biotechnology-based production of Shiitake and other exotic mushrooms. The company employs patented processes to produce an extensive range of quality mushrooms and mushroom nutraceutical products.

12 SciencePark Drive #04-01, The Mendel Singapore Science Park 1

Singapore 118225

Phone: +65 6773-0377

Fax: +65 6773-1766

Email: info@mycobiotech.com

Website: http://www.mycobiotech.com

Tekoa Mushroom Farm (Israel)

Tekoa group differs from others in its customized approach to the design and operation of mushroom farms and processing facilities and its consistent focus on commercial/economic factors. It specializes in shiitake mushrooms.

Mobile Post North Judea, 90908, Israel

Phone: +972 2 9964527

Fax: +972 2 9964588

Website: http://www.tekoafarms.co.il/index1.htm

E-mail: ok@tekoafarms.co.il

Organizations

Australasian Mycological Society

Website: bugs.bio.usyd.edu.au/AustMycolSoc/Home/ams.html

Korean Society of Mycology

Website: www.mycology.or.kr/english/index.asp

Mycological Society of Japan

Website: www.coara.or.jp/~murakami/html/index-e.html

AFRICA

Sources for Mushrooms and Mushroom Supplements

Nature's Gift for Life (Cameroon)
Bonadouma Home, Bonapriso, Douala, Cameroon
Phone: + 237 785-6155
Website: ng4lnutritionals.com
E-mail: sales@ng4lnutritionals.com

Cili Health (South Africa)
Cili Health Pty, SA, distributes a full line of US made, Certified Organic medicinal mushroom medicines throughout the countries of southern Africa. All Cili Health products have been approved as 'Complementary Medicines' by the South African Medicines Council, so they can be (and are!) used in hospitals and clinics; they are prescribed by doctors and are paid for by health insurance. Cili Health is also providing meals for the school lunch feeding program in the Kingdom of Swaziland, which includes a US-manufactured medicinal mushroom formulation for helping combat the effects of HIV infection.
Corporate: Life Enrichment Centre, 100 Main Road, Newlands, Johannesburg
Mailing address: P.O. Box 69956, Bryanston 2021, South Africa
Phone: ++27 11 477-9429
Website: www.cili-bao.co.za
E-mail: sales@cili-bao.co.za

Lifestyle Nutrition Products (South Africa)
Lifestyle Nutrition Products manufacture their own line of medicinal mushroom-based performance products, distributed throughout South Africa and very popular with the footballer crowd and other professional athletes. *Cordyceps* may well be one of the reasons South Africa wins so many football (soccer) matches! Lifestyle's formulations are all made using USDA Certified Organic materials, grown in the US and tableted in South Africa.
Eastdale Pavilion, 649 Vercueil Street, Garsfontein, Pretoria 0042, South Africa
Phone: ++27 12 998-9770
Website: www.lifestylenp.com

SOUTH AMERICA

Sources for Mushrooms and Mushroom Supplements

Agaricus RBBZ Imports & Exports *(Agaricus blazei)* (Brazil)
SCS Qd. 06 Ed. Jose Severo, Sobrejola 02, Brasilia DF, Brasil

Mushroom Recipes

Some of the mushrooms described in this book, maitake and shiitake especially, are delicious, so try your hand at using them in soups, stir-fry dishes, and stews. When you do so, however, be sure to cook them in such a way that they keep their nutrients. The rules that apply to cooking vegetables also apply to cooking mushrooms. If you want to keep the mushrooms' nutrients, you must recover the water in which they are cooked, as the beta-glucans in mushrooms dissolve into cooking water. Likewise, many nutrients dissolve into the cooking oil when you stir-fry mushrooms. What's more, overcooking depletes the mushrooms of some of their nutrients.

The best way to prepare mushrooms is to include the cooking liquids in the dish you are preparing and be careful not to cook the mushrooms for too long. Some connoisseurs believe in tearing mushrooms instead of cutting them to preserve nutrients. By tearing, the mushroom pieces are separated along the cell walls.

To clean mushrooms, trim the bottom of the stems and then wipe off the mushrooms. *Do not* soak or rinse them. Mushrooms absorb water, so if you wash them in water, they will turn soggy and lose some of their crispness and flavor.

Of course, you can always rely on medicinal mushroom powders and capsules to get nutrients from mushrooms. If you prefer not to take powders and capsules, try mixing them into soups or baking them into breads. By the way, mixing medicinal mushroom powders into food is an excellent way to give medicinal mushrooms to children, who often balk at taking pills and capsules.

149

MAITAKE

The Hen of the Woods is a delicacy. The Japanese would pay more than the French spend on truffles for a large *Grifola frondosa*. Maitakes have an amazing taste: the rich, woodsy flavor and the firm, meaty texture of the flesh make them the standout ingredient of any dish. Maitakes are on their way to becoming one of the staples of the Asian diet (along with soy, fish, and tea) since they confer "good health and longevity." Florence Fabricant, the food editor of *The New York Times,* says the maitake mushroom is "quite meaty, with a delicately nutty flavor, and holds its shape and crisp texture extremely well in the sauté pan. And it doesn't sop as much oil as other mushrooms." Their unique aroma and crunchy texture make maitakes a perfect match for any type of cuisine. And being rich in vitamins B1, B2, and D, as well as vegetable fiber and polysaccharides, maitake mushrooms promote good health.

MAITAKE CHAWAN MUSHI

Chawan Mushi is a popular Japanese egg custard dish. In fact, special China cups are made for preparing and serving the custard. The cups come with lids that are used to keep the custard warm for a while after it is served. Here, in Chef Ming Tsai's recipe, ramekins have been substituted for the traditional cups.

2-1/2 cups dashi* (may substitute vegetable stock)

3 eggs

1 tbsp soy sauce (naturally brewed)

1/2 cup maitake mushroom petals

1 tbsp scallions, thinly sliced

Grapeseed oil

Salt and pepper (to taste)

4 small ramekins or tea cups

*Dashi is the traditional Japanese stock. It is prepared with konbu, a nutritious seaweed, and flakes of dried bonito, a fish that's long been a staple of the Japanese diet. If you are short on time, you can use dashi powder to make the stock. Just look for brands that contain no monosodium glutamate (MSG).

To prepare dashi, you will need one piece (about 5–6 inches) of konbu and 1 cup of bonito flakes. Clean the konbu by wiping it with a damp cloth. Then place it in a stockpot with 5 cups of cold water and heat over medium heat. Just before the water boils, remove it from the heat. Watch carefully—you do not want the water to boil or the dashi will become too strongly flavored. Allow to stand 5 minutes, remove the konbu and return the pot to medium heat. When the stock once again nears the boiling point, remove the pot from the heat and add the bonito flakes. When the flakes sink to the bottom of the pot, strain the dashi through cheesecloth or a fine-mesh strainer.

Directions: In a large bowl, whisk together the dashi, eggs, and soy sauce. Season with the salt and pepper (to taste). Skim the bubbles and the foam off the top. Heat a medium skillet over high heat, then add the oil and swirl to coat the pan. When the oil shimmers, add the maitakes and sauté until soft, about 6 minutes. Season to taste with salt and pepper. Evenly divide the cooked maitakes among the ramekins and sprinkle with the scallions.

Fill the ramekins with 4 oz of the egg mixture, making sure not to create any bubbles. Place the ramekin in a hot water bath and cover with aluminum foil. Fill a metal pan with enough boiling water so that the water goes halfway up the side of the ramekin. Place the pan in a 375°F oven for 5 minutes, then reduce the heat to 325°F and cook for another 15–20 minutes.

(From Ming's Pantry, http://www.mingspantry.com/maitmuschawm.html.)

MAITAKE RICE PILAF

2 cups long-grain white/brown rice
(a little wild rice mixed in is good too), washed and uncooked
4 cups chicken or bean stock
1 cup lentils, cooked
2–3 cups maitake mushrooms, chopped
1 cup onions, coarsely chopped
1 cup celery, coarsely chopped
2 cloves garlic, minced
1 cup peanuts or almonds, chopped
1 tbsp parsley
1 tbsp allspice
3 tbsp olive oil
Salt, pepper, cayenne pepper (to taste)

In a large saucepan, sauté mushrooms and garlic in olive oil over medium-high heat for 15 minutes, adding parsley, onions, celery, and pepper after 10 minutes. Add rice and stir for another 3 minutes, then add stock, lentils, allspice, and salt. Stir again, then let sit until mixture is boiling gently. Reduce heat and cover; simmer for 20 minutes, then check mixture. If all of the liquid has been reduced by that time, add ½ cup extra liquid (stock, sherry, soy sauce, etc.), salt, cayenne pepper to taste, peanuts/almonds, and then cook for 15 more minutes. Let cool uncovered for 5 minutes and serve with a dollop of plain yogurt on top.

TWICE-BAKED POTATOES WITH MAITAKE MUSHROOMS AND SMOKY GOUDA

4 large baking potatoes (baked until almost cooked through)
6 oz smoky gouda, grated
½ stick of butter
2 oz maitake mushrooms (dried)
3–4 slices pancetta or bacon, diced

Cut potatoes lengthwise in half. Scoop out potato into a bowl and try not to damage the skins. Add 6 oz grated smoky gouda and ½ stick of butter to the warm potato and smash a little. Reconstitute 2 oz of maitake mushroom in hot tap water for 15 minutes. Drain, chop, put in a small skillet with 3–4 slices of pancetta or bacon, diced. Sauté until the bacon is crisp. Combine this with the potato mixture and scoop it back into the potato skins. Top with a little gouda and bake again until hot.

SHIITAKE

There are dozens of cookbooks devoted to the bounty and flavors of *Lentinula edodes,* not to mention hundreds of tempting recipes available online. Shop with care when purchasing dried shiitakes, since there are many grades and prices. The caps may be thick and fleshy or thin, large or small, cracked on top or smooth. The very thick, cracked-topped *donko* types are expensive, but worth the price. They are meaty and can stand up to any food flavors.

Because shiitakes grow on wood or other coarse cellulose materials, the fresh mushrooms are very clean. Brush the caps lightly. As a rule, the stems are tough, so cut them off using a knife or scissors. The stems can be used to add flavor to a stock.

Lentinula edodes will enhance the flavor of most foods, except, perhaps, baked ham. It is also tasty by itself, cooked several different ways. It accents vegetables, meats, seafood, poultry, and even other mushrooms. The classic way of handling dried caps is to simmer them in water with a little soy sauce to make a shiitake bouillon. Added to a light cream sauce, the shiitake is ideal for flavoring pasta dishes.

Reconstitute dried mushrooms by soaking in hot or boiling water for 20 minutes. Save the liquid to include with your food for another dish. Pour off the liquid at the top to separate it from any debris at the bottom of the dish in which it was soaked.

STEAMED STUFFED SHIITAKES

24 large dried shiitakes, stems removed
½ pound ground lean pork
1 green onion, sliced fine
1 small slice fresh ginger, peeled and minced
2 tbsp soy sauce
1 tbsp dry sherry
1 egg white, slightly beaten
1 tbsp cornstarch
1 tbsp fresh cilantro, chopped

Prepare these mushrooms in a container that fits into a steamer. Save the rich juice and pour it over white rice. Soak the mushrooms for 15 minutes in hot water to cover. Drain and squeeze dry; reserve the soaking liquid. Mix the pork, green onion, ginger, soy sauce, sherry, egg white, and cornstarch. Mound the stuffing into the mushroom caps. Place in a heatproof dish that will fit into your steamer. Steam for 20–25 minutes. Toss the cilantro on top. Serves 12 as an appetizer.

SPINACH AND SHIITAKE SALAD WITH CITRUS DRESSING

1 package (3-½ ounces) shiitake mushrooms
6 cups spinach leaves, trimmed in bite-sized pieces
and lightly-packed
1 cup tomatoes, chopped
¼ cup grapefruit juice
¼ cup vegetable oil
½ tsp Dijon-style prepared mustard
¼ tsp salt
⅛ tsp black pepper, ground

Trim stem ends of shiitake mushrooms, then cut into thin slices, through the caps and stems. In a large serving bowl, place the mushrooms, spinach, and tomatoes; set aside. In a small bowl, whisk together grapefruit juice, oil, mustard, salt, and pepper. Just before serving, pour over the vegetables, tossing gently. Makes 4 portions.

REISHI

Ganoderma lucidum is very bitter and tough, but because reishi has unsurpassed medicinal benefits, it is worth considering these two original Chinese recipes.

Brewing Reishi

Cut up the dried reishi into small pieces, the smaller the better. For a daily portion, take 3–5 grams (g) of mushrooms, add 3 bowls of water (about 600 cc), and boil for 30 minutes using low heat. Only use clay pots or glassware; avoid the use of metallic containers. The boiled reishi can be used again until the bitter taste is gone; usually, it is good for 2–3 uses. You can prepare 2–3 days worth at one time and keep it in the refrigerator for daily use. Reheat before use, and it is best to drink before each meal. For people with stomach problems, drink the brew after each meal. If you dislike the brew's bitter taste, add pure honey or glucose (avoid the use of refined sugar).

You can also mix reishi pieces with brandy or Chinese wine; store for 3–4 months before use. Reishi should be stored in a cool, dry place, but never in the refrigerator. Note: Used reishi pieces can be used as a fertilizer for house plants.

REISHI SOUP

10 g reishi pieces, sliced
6 whole quails, frozen or fresh
70 g dry scallops
100 g pork, lean
3 pints (1.5 liter) hot water
Salt and pepper (to taste)
Dash cooking wine

Soak the sliced reishi pieces in 3 pints of water for 4 hours. Remove the quails from boiling water after 5 seconds and put in a Chinese steam pot. Pour in the 3 pints of water together with the reishi pieces. Add dry scallops, pork, and a dash of cooking wine. Steam boil for 3 hours. Before use, season the soup with salt and pepper, according to taste.

Note: You can add dried long-gang meat or dry red dates to sweeten the soup. You can also substitute 2 frozen whole pigeons, a whole chicken, or half a turtle instead of the 6 quails for the above recipe.

REISHI TEA

1 tsp dried reishi, chopped
7 thin slices ginger root, fresh
1 cup water

Combine the ingredients in a small pan. Bring to a boil, then simmer for 10 minutes or so. Strain the tea and enjoy!

CORDYCEPS SINENSIS

Wild *Cordyceps* is usually consumed as part of an elaborate soup or stew. The following recipe comes from the kitchens of the Ming emperors.

CHICKEN SOUP WITH *ASTRAGALUS*, GINSENG, *CORDYCEPS*, AND DATES

1–2 tbsp sesame oil, organic cold-pressed
3–4 slices ginger root, fresh
1 medium brown onion, sliced
1–2 cups root vegetables of your choice (carrot, turnip, rutabaga, daikon), chopped
2–3 chicken legs (or other parts if you like), skinless and hormone-free
1 tbsp dark miso paste
1 tsp white pepper (more or less to taste)

HERBS:
2–3 oz *Astragalus* root (Huang Qi)
1 oz Chinese red ginseng root (Ren Shen)
1 oz American ginseng root (Xi Yang Shen)
5–6 pieces *Cordyceps* fungus (Dong Chong Xia Cao)
3 pieces *Dioscorea* yam root (Shan Yao)
1–2 pieces aged tangerine peel (Chen Pi)
3–4 pieces Chinese red date (Da Zao)
2–3 Indian green cardamon pods or Chinese cardamon (Sha Ren)
3–4 pieces *Poria* fungus (Fu Ling)

Fry the sliced brown onion and thinly sliced ginger root in the sesame oil. When slightly browned, add as much chicken as you like. Vegetarians may substitute tofu or tempeh at this stage. Sauté for 5 minutes longer and then add the root vegetables and herbs with enough water to reach 2–3 inches above the ingredients. Bring to a boil and reduce to medium-low. Cook for 45 minutes to 1 hour in a heavy pot with a tight lid. Ten minutes before finishing, add the miso paste (after mixing it in a little water) and the pepper and let it simmer to perfection. Salt can be added if the miso is not salty enough. Those on a low-fat diet can reduce the oil to 1 tsp, but generally fat is not the issue for those eating this soup.

Cordyceps Duck

Here is a traditional Chinese recipe for preparing *Cordyceps* Duck:

Cordyceps sinensis (12 grams)
1 duck (750 grams)
White wine (dash)
Scallions (2 tablespoons)
Chicken stock (1 quart)
Ginger (1 tablespoon)

Soak the *Cordyceps* in lukewarm water until it is soft. Meanwhile, boil the duck thoroughly. Place the duck in a new pot along with the cooking wine, scallions, soup stock, and ginger. Add salt. Seal the pot tightly and steam for three hours. When done, remove the ginger and scallions. Add pepper.

AGARICUS BLAZEI

Agaricus blazei is a delicious medical mushroom. It is often called an almond portobello mushroom because of its strong almond flavor.

"ALMOND PORTOBELLO" MUSHROOMS WITH ALMOND-BULGUR STUFFING

1 cup bulgur wheat

$\frac{1}{2}$ cup onion, diced

1-$\frac{1}{2}$ cups water

1 can (14-$\frac{1}{2}$ ounces) vegetable broth, divided

Salt

1 tsp thyme, dried

Pepper

1 jar (15 oz) roasted red peppers (about 2 cups), divided

$\frac{1}{2}$ cup fresh whole-wheat bread crumbs (1 slice)

$\frac{1}{2}$ cup almonds, sliced and toasted

$\frac{1}{4}$ cup parsley, chopped

1 tbsp lemon juice

2 tbsp balsamic vinegar

4 (5–6 inch) *Agaricus blazei*

("almond portobello") mushroom caps

To make the stuffing, heat 1–$\frac{1}{2}$ tsp oil in a 3-quart saucepan over medium heat. Add bulgur and onion and sauté until the onion is translucent and the bulgur is toasted. Add water, 1–$\frac{1}{2}$ cups broth, 1 tsp salt, the thyme and $\frac{1}{4}$ teaspoon pepper. Cover and bring to a boil; lower heat and simmer about 15 minutes until liquid is almost gone. Chop enough of the peppers to make $\frac{1}{2}$ cup; reserve remaining peppers. Mix chopped peppers, crumbs, almonds, parsley, and juice into bulgur mixture; keep warm.

To make the sauce, in a blender, pulse remaining peppers and broth, the vinegar and $\frac{1}{4}$ tsp salt until smooth.

Heat griddle or grill over medium-high heat. Brush mushroom caps with oil and season with salt and pepper. Cook 5 minutes, then turn over and continue to cook about 5 minutes until tender. Divide stuffing among four plates. Slice mushrooms and fan over stuffing. Spoon sauce around edges. Garnish with additional toasted sliced almonds, if desired. Makes 4 servings.

Note: To make fresh bread crumbs, place quartered bread slice into a food processor. Pulse on and off until bread is ground into crumbs.

GRILLED "ALMOND PORTOBELLO" MUSHROOMS AND VEGGIE FAJITAS

3 tbsp balsamic vinegar

3 tbsp olive oil

2 tbsp parsley, freshly chopped

1 tbsp garlic, minced

¼ tsp salt

⅛ tsp black pepper, freshly ground

4 medium almond portobello mushrooms, washed well and patted dry

2 red onions, sliced

2 red or orange peppers, destemmed, deseeded,
and cut into quarters lengthwise

2 green peppers, destemmed, deseeded,
and cut into quarters lengthwise

2 jalapeno peppers, destemmed, deseeded,
and cut in half lengthwise

4–8 inch flour tortillas

In a large bowl, place the vinegar, olive oil, parsley, garlic, salt, and pepper, and whisk well to combine. Add all of the vegetables and toss to thoroughly coat the vegetables with the marinade. Set the vegetables aside and allow them to marinate for 15 minutes. Place the vegetables on a hot grill for 3–5 minutes per side or until tender. (The vegetables can also be cooked under the broiler for 3–5 minutes per side or until tender.) Transfer the grilled vegetables to a cutting board and cut them into strips. The tortillas can be warmed on the grill, if desired. Transfer the vegetables to a platter for serving. Allow guests to build their own fajitas by filling tortillas with the grilled vegetables. Makes 4 servings.

PHELLINUS LINTEUS

Phellinus linteus has a hard wooden texture and saws or knives are needed to chop it into small pieces. The Koreans recommend taking the mushroom three times a day regularly: early in the morning, with lunch, and after dinner (3–6 grams each time). The following recipe is a popular one.

MULBERRY YELLOW POLYPORE

30 g *Phellinus linteus* mushrooms

Water

Place *Phellinus linteus* mushrooms and 1.8 liter water in a pot, and set it to boil. When boiling starts, lower the heat and let it simmer until the water is reduced to about 1.5 liter. Drain the liquid into a bowl. Add 1.2 liter of water to the pot, bring it to a boil, and let it simmer until the water is reduced to 0.9 liter. Drain the liquid into the bowl (i.e., mix the liquids). Dry the mushrooms and mix them with rice wine and you will enjoy a wonderful medicinal drink! Drink the liquid three times a day.

HERICIUM ERINACEUS

An unusual and beautiful mushroom, *Hericium erinaceus* (lion's mane mushroom) takes on a crab-like flavor when sautéed in butter. Store fresh lion's mane mushrooms in a paper bag in the refrigerator for up to seven days. Dried mushrooms should be stored in a tightly sealed container, in a cool, dry place. It grows yellow and sour-tasting with age, so buy only white ones. *Hericium erinaceus* can be sautéed, broiled, grilled, or added to any recipe that requires mushrooms. They are especially tasty when served over fish or combined with fresh vegetables.

CHARLENE'S QUICHE

1 pastry shell

1-$\frac{1}{2}$ cups cheese, grated

1 medium onion, diced

$\frac{1}{2}$ pound lion's mane mushrooms, sliced

1 tbsp butter

1 tbsp olive oil

Dash salt and pepper

1 cup milk

2 tbsp flour

$\frac{1}{4}$ tsp dry mustard

3 eggs

Cover bottom of pastry shell with cheese. Sauté mushrooms and onion in a mixture of 1 tbsp butter and 1 tbsp olive oil until softened. Place mushroom/onion mixture on top of cheese. Add salt and pepper to taste. Beat together the flour, eggs, milk, and dry mustard and pour over the mushroom layer. Bake at 375°F for 45 minutes or until the center is firm. Hint: Use the mushrooms at their peak, when they are white and firm. (From *The Mushroom Growers' Newsletter*)

References

Chapter 1

Arora, D. *Mushrooms Demystified: A Comprehensive Guide to Fleshy Fungi*. Berkeley, CA: Ten Speed Press, 1986.

Schaechter, E. *In the Company of Mushrooms*. Cambridge, MA: Harvard University Press, 1997.

Schaechter, E. "Weird and Wonderful Fungi." *Microbiol Today* 27 (2000): 116–117.

Smith, M.L., et al. "The Fungus, *Armarillaria bulbosa*, is Among the Largest and Oldest Living Organisms." *Nature* 356 (1992): 428–431.

Wasser, S.P. "Review of Medicinal Mushroom Advances: Good News from Old Allies." *HerbalGram* 56 (2002): 28–33.

Chapter 2

Beinfield, H., et al. "Chinese Traditional Medicine: An Introductory Overview." *Altern Ther* 1 (1995): 44–52.

Berman, B., et al. *Alternative Medicine: Expanding Medical Horizons*. NIH Publication No. 94-166. Bethesda, MD: National Institutes of Health, 1994.

Hobbs, C. *Medicinal Mushrooms: An Exploration of Tradition, Healing, and Culture*. Santa Cruz, CA: Botanica Press, 1986.

Huddler, G. *Magical Mushrooms, Mischievous Molds*. Princeton, NJ: Princeton University Press, 1998.

Kaptchuck, T. *The Web That Has No Weaver: Understanding Chinese Medicine*. Chicago: Contemporary Books, 2000.

Keys, J. *Chinese Herbs: Their Botany, Chemistry, and Pharmacodynamics*. Rutland, VT: Charles E. Tuttle, 1998.

Lindequist, U., et al. "Neue Wirtstoffe aus Basidiomyceten." *Z Phytoter* 11 (1990): 139–149.

Lindequist, U., et al. "The Pharmacological Potential of Mushrooms." *eCAM* 2 (2005): 285–299.

Nakagaki, T. "Intelligence: Maze-solving by an Amoeboid Organism." *Nature* 407 (2000): 123–125.

Spindler, K. *The Man in the Ice: The Discovery of a 5,000-Year-Old Body Reveals the Secrets of the Stone Age.* New York: Bantam Books, 1994.

Upton, H. "Origin of Drugs in Current Use: The Cyclosporin Story." Available online at: http://www.world-of-fungi.org/Mostly_Medical/Harriet_Upton/Harriet_Upton.htm.

Wasson, R. Gordon. *The Divine Mushroom of Immortality.* New York: Harcourt Brace Jovanovich, 1968.

Yue, D., et al. *Advanced Study for Traditional Chinese Herbal Medicine, Institute of Materia Medica.* Beijing, China: Medical University and China Peking Union Medical University Press, 1995.

Chapter 3

Adachi, Y., et al. "The Effect Enhancement of Cytokine Production by Macrophages Stimulated with 1,3 Beta-D-glucan, Grifolan, Isolated from *Grifola frondosa*." *Biol Pharm Bull* 17 (1994): 1554–1560.

Browder, I.W., et al. "Beneficial Effect of Enhanced Macrophage Function in Trauma Patients." *Ann Surg* 211 (1990): 605–613.

Cancer Research UK. "Medicinal Mushrooms and Cancer." Available online at: http://www.sci.cancerresearchuk.org/labs/med_mush/med_mush.html.

Clute, M. "Beta-glucan: The Little Branched-chain Polysaccharide that Might." *Natural Foods Merchandiser* 3 (2001): 21–24.

DiLuzio, N. "Immunopharmacology of Glucan: A Broad-spectrum Enhancer of Host Defense Mechanisms." *Trends Pharmacol* 4 (1983): 344–347.

Gibson, G., et al. "Dietary Modulation of the Human Colonic Microbiota: Introducing the Concept of Prebiotics." *J Nutr* 125 (1995): 1401–1412.

Lewis, R. "Portals for Prions? Investigators Look at a Potential Pathway for Prions." *The Scientist.* 7 (2001): 1.

Lui, E. "Free Radical Scavenging Activities of Mushroom Polysaccharide Extracts." *Life Sci* 60:10 (1997): 763–771.

Manfreds, D., et al. "Morbidity and Mortality from Chronic Obstructive Pulmonary Disease." *Ann Rev Resp Dis* 140 (1992): S19–S26.

Mansell, P.W., et al. "Macrophage-mediated Destruction of Human Malignant Cells *in vivo.*" *J Natl Cancer Inst* 54 (1975): 571–580.

Martensen, R. "Cancer: Medical History and the Framing of a Disease." *JAMA* 271 (1994): 24–28.

Mizuno, T., et al. "Health Foods and Medicinal Usage of Mushrooms." *Food Rev Intern* 11 (1995): 69–81.

Ohno, N., et al. "Effect of Beta-glucan on the Nitric Oxide Synthesis of Peritoneal Macrophage in Mice." *Biol Pharm Bull* 19 (1996): 608–612.

Ooi, V.E.C., et al. "A Review of Pharmacological Activities of Mushroom Polysaccharides." *Int J Med Mushr* 1 (1999): 195–206.

Raa, J., et al. "The Use of Immunostimulants to Increase Resistance of Aquatic Organisms to Microbial Infection." *J Dermatol Surg Oncol* 15 (1989): 1199–1202.

Reshetnikov, S.C., et al. "Higher *Basidiomycetes* as a Source of Antitumour and Immunostimulating Polysaccharides." *Int J Med Mushr* 3 (2001): 361–394.

Rodman, W.L. "Cancer: Its Etiology and Treatment." *Am Pract News* 16 (1893): 409–417.

Ross, G.D., et al. "Therapeutic Intervention with Complement and Beta-glucan in Cancer." *Immunopharmacology* 42 (1999): 61–74.

Sharon, N., et al. "Carbohydrates in Cell Recognition." *Scient Am J* (1993): 74–81.

Wasser, S.P., et al. "Medicinal Properties of Substances Occurring in Higher *Basidiomycete* Mushrooms: Current Perspectives." *Int J Med Mushr* 1 (1999): 31–62.

Wasser, S.P. "Review of Medicinal Mushroom Advances: Good News from Old Allies." *HerbalGram* 56 (2002): 28–33.

Chapter 4

Adachi, Y., et al. "Enhancement of Cytokine Production by Macrophages Stimulated with 1-3 Beta-D-glucan, Grifolan (GRN), Isolated from *Grifola frondosa.*" *Biol Pharm Bull* 17 (1994): 1554–1560.

Andrioli, G., et al. "Differential Effects of Dietary Supplementation with Fish Oil or Soy Lecithin on Human Platelet Adhesion." *Thromb Haemost* 82 (1999): 1522–1527.

Appel, L.J., et al. "DASH Collaborative Research Group: A Clinical Trial of the Effects of Dietary Patterns on Blood Pressure." *N Engl J Med* 336 (1997): 1117–1124.

Avula, B., et al. "Determination of the Appetite Suppressant P57 in *Hoodia gordonii* Plant Extracts and Dietary Supplements by Liquid Chromatography/Electrospray Ionization Mass Spectrometry (LC-MSD-TOF) and LC-UV Methods." *J AOAC Int* 89:3 (2006): 606–611.

Cancer Research UK. "Medicinal Mushrooms and Cancer." Available online at: http://www.sci.cancerresearchuk.org/labs/med_mush/med_mush.html.

Chopra, M., et al. "Antioxidants and Lipoprotein Metabolism." *Proc Nutr Soc* 58 (1999): 663–671.

Collene, A.L., et al. "Effects of a Nutritional Supplement Containing *Salacia oblonga* Extract and Insulinogenic Amino Acids on Postprandial Glycemia, Insulinemia, and Breath Hydrogen Responses in Healthy Adults." *Nutrition* 21:7–8 (2005): 848–854.

Fullerton, S.A., et al. "Induction of Apoptosis in Human Prostatic Cancer Cells with Beta-glucan (Maitake Mushroom Polysaccharide)." *Mol Urol* 4 (2000): 7–13.

Giroux, I., et al. "Addition of Arginine but not Glycine to Lysine plus Methionine-enriched Diets Modulates Serum Cholesterol and Liver Phospholipids in Rabbits." *J Nutr* 129 (1999): 1807–1313.

Hare, J.T., et al. "Grapefruit Juice and Potential Drug Interactions." *Consul Pharm* 18:5 (2003): 466–472.

Horio, H., et al. "Maitake (*Grifola frondosa*) Improves Glucose Tolerance of Experimental Diabetic Rats." *J Nutr Sci Vitaminol (Tokyo)* 47:1 (2001): 57–63.

Huang, T.H., et al. "*Salacia oblonga* Root Improves Cardiac Lipid Metabolism in Zucker Diabetic Fatty Rats: Modulation of Cardiac PPAR-alpha-mediated Transcription of Fatty Acid Metabolic Genes." *Toxicol Appl Pharmacol* 210:1–2 (2006): 78-85.

Jenkins, D.J., et al. "Viscous and Nonviscous Fibres, Nonabsorbable and Low Glycaemic Index Carbohydrates, Blood Lipids and Coronary Heart Disease." *Curr Opin Lipidol* 11 (2000): 49–56.

Jones, K. "Maitake: A Potent Medicinal Food." *Alt Comp Ther* 4 (1998): 420–429.

Khan, A., et al. "Cinnamon Improves Glucose and Lipids of People with Type 2 Diabetes." *Diabetes Care* 26:12 (2003): 3215–3218.

Klurfeld, D.M. "Synergy Between Medical and Nutrient Therapies: George Washington meets Rodney Dangerfield." *J Am Coll Nutr* 20:5 Suppl (2001): 349S-353S.

Kodama, N., A. Asakawa, A. Inui, et al. "Enhancement of Cytotoxicity of NK Cells by D-fraction, a Polysaccharide from *Grifola frondosa*." *Oncol Rep* 13:3 (2005): 497–502.

Kodama, N., et al. "Can Maitake MD-fraction Aid Cancer Patients?" *Alt Med Rev* 7:3 (2002): 236–239.

Krauss, R.M., et al. "AHA Dietary Guidelines Revision 2000: A Statement for

Healthcare Professionals from the Nutrition Committee of the American Heart Association." *Circulation* 102 (2000): 2284–2299.

Kubo, K., et al. "Anti-diabetic Activity Present in the Fruit-body of *Grifola fron-dosa* (Maitake)." *Biol Pharm Bull* 17 (1994): 1106–1110.

Kubo, K., et al. "The Effect of Maitake Mushrooms on Liver and Serum Lipids." *Altern Ther Health Med* 2 (1996): 62–66.

Kuhn, D., et al. "Synthetic Peracetate Tea Polyphenols as Potent Proteasome Inhibitors and Apoptosis Inducers in Human Cancer Cells." *Front Biosci* 10 (2005): 1010–1023.

Kurashige, S., et al. "Effects of *Lentinus edodes, Grifola frondosa* and *Pleurotus ostreatus* Administration on Cancer Outbreak, and Activities of Macrophages and Lymphocytes in Mice Treated with a Carcinogen, Nbutyl-N-butanolni-trosoamine." *Immunopharmacol Immunotoxicol* 19 (1997): 175–183.

Landis-Piwowar, K.R., et al. "Evaluation of Proteasome-inhibitory and Apopto-sis-inducing Potencies of Novel (-)-EGCG Analogs and their Prodrugs." *Int J Mol Med* 15:4 (2005): 735–742.

Lee, E.W., et al. "Suppression of D-galactosamine-induced Liver Injury by Mush-rooms in Rats." *Biosci Biotechnol Biochem* 64 (2000): 2001–2004.

Mang, B., et al. "Effects of a Cinnamon Extract on Plasma Glucose, HbA, and Serum Lipids in Diabetes Mellitus Type 2." *Eur J Clin Invest* 36:5 (2006): 340–344.

Mann, J.I. "Can Dietary Intervention Produce Long-term Reduction in Insulin Resistance?" *Br J Nutr* 83:Suppl 1 (2000): 169S–172S.

Martin, J., et al. "Chromium Picolinate Supplementation Attenuates Body Weight Gain and Increases Insulin Sensitivity in Subjects with Type 2 Diabetes." *Diabetes Care* 29:8 (2006): 1826–1832.

Mayell, M. "Maitake Extracts and Their Therapeutic Potential." *Altern Med Rev* 6:1 (2001): 48–60.

Mizuno, T., et al. "Maitake, *Grifola frondosa:* Pharmacological Effects." *Food Rev Intl* 11 (1995): 135–149.

Nakai, R., et al. "Effect of Maitake (*Grifola frondosa*) Water Extract on Inhibition of Adipocyte Conversion of C3H10T$^1/_2$B2C1 Cells." *J Nutr Sci Vitaminol (Tokyo)* 45 (1999): 385–390.

Nanba, H. "Maitake D-fraction: Healing and Preventive Potential for Cancer." *J Orthomol Med* 12 (1997): 43–49.

Nanba, H., et al. "Effects of Maitake (*Grifola frondosa*) Glucan in HIV-infected Patients." *Mycoscience* 41 (2000): 293–295.

Nishida, I., et al. "Antitumour Activity Exhibited by Orally Administered

Extracts from Fruit-body of *Grifola frondosa* (Maitake)." *Chem Pharmac Bull* 36 (1988): 1819–1827.

Ohno, N., et al. "Enhancement of LPS Triggered TNF-alpha (Tumor Necrosis Factor-alpha) Production by 1-3 Beta-D-glucan in Mice." *Biol Pharm Bull* 18 (1995): 126–133.

Ohtsuru, M. "Anti-obesity Activity Exhibited by Orally Administered Powder of Maitake Mushroom (*Grifola frondosa*)." *Anshin* 7 (1992): 198–200.

Okazaki, M., et al. "Structure-activity Relationship of 1-3 Beta-D-glucans in the Induction of Cytokine Production from Macrophages, *in vitro*." *Biol Pharm Bull* 18 (1995): 1320–1327.

Pattar, G.R., et al. "Chromium Picolinate Positively Influences the Glucose Transporter System via Affecting Cholesterol Homeostasis in Adipocytes Cultured Under Hyperglycemic Diabetic Conditions." *Mutat Res* (July 24, 2006); Epub ahead of print.

Pei, D., et al. "The Influence of Chromium Chloride-containing Milk to Glycemic Control of Patients with Type 2 Diabetes Mellitus: A Randomized, Double-blind, Placebo-controlled Trial." *Metabolism* 55:7 (2006): 923–927.

Riccardi, G., et al. "Dietary Treatment of the Metabolic Syndrome—The Optimal Diet." *Br J Nutr* 83:Suppl 1 (2000): 143S–148S.

Svetkey, L.P., et al., for the DASH Research Group. "Effects of Dietary Patterns on Blood Pressure. Subgroup Analysis of the Dietary Approaches to Stop Hypertension (DASH) Randomized Clinical Trial." *Arch Intern Med* 159 (1999): 285–293.

Tsao, P.S., et al. "L-arginine Attenuates Platelet Reactivity in Hypercholesterolemic Rabbits." *Arterioscler Thromb* 14 (1994): 1529–1533.

Yokota, M. "Observatory Trial of Anti-obesity Activity of Maitake (*Grifola frondosa*)." *Anshin* 7 (1992): 202–204.

Zhang, Y., et al. "Cyclooxygenase Inhibitory and Antioxidant Compounds from the Mycelia of the Edible Mushroom *Grifola frondosa*." *J Agric Food Chem* 50:26 (2002): 7581–7585.

Zhuang, C., et al. "Biological Responses from *Grifola frondosa* (Dick.:Fr.) S.F. Gray-Maitake (Aphyllophormycetideaea)." *Int J Med Mushr* 1 (1999): 317–324.

Chapter 5

Akamatsu, S., et al. "Hepatoprotective Effect of Extracts from *Lentinus edodes* Mycelia on Dimethylnitrosamine-induced Liver Injury." *Biol Pharm Bull* 27:12 (2004): 1957–1960.

Amagase, H. "Treatment of Hepatitis B Patients with *Lentinula edodes* Mycelium." Proceedings XII International Congress on Gastroenterology, Lisbon, Portugal, 1987, p. 197.

Bae, E.A., et al. "Effect of *Lentinus edodes* on the Growth of Intestinal Lactic Acid Bacteria." *Arch Pharmac Res* 20 (1997): 443–447.

Bender, S., et al. "A Case for Caution in Assessing the Antibiotic Activity of Extracts of Culinary-medicinal Shiitake Mushroom [*Lentinus edodes* (Berk.) Singer] (Agaricomycetidae)." *Int J Med Mushr* 5 (2003): 31–35.

Bratkovich, S.M. "Shiitake Mushroom Production: Obtaining Spawn, Obtaining and Preparing Logs, and Inoculation." Available online at: http://ohioline.osu.edu/for-fact/0040.html.

Cancer Research UK. "Medicinal Mushrooms and Cancer." Available online at: http://www.sci.cancerresearchuk.org/labs/med_mush/med_mush.html.

Chihara, G., et al. "Fractionation and Purification of the Polysaccharides with Marked Anti-tumor Activity, Especially Lentinan from *Lentinus edodes* (Berk.) Sing., an Edible Mushroom." *Cancer Res* 30 (1970): 2776–2781.

Gadek, J.E., et al. "Effect of Enteral Feeding with Eicosapentaenoic Acid, Gamma-linolenic Acid, and Antioxidants in Patients with Acute Respiratory Distress Syndrome. Enteral Nutrition in ARDS Study Group." *Crit Care Med* 27 (1999): 1409–1420.

Gordon, M., et al. "A Placebo-controlled Trial of the Immune Modulator, Lentinan, in HIV-positive Patients: A Phase I/II Trial." *J Med* 29 (1998): 305–330.

Hatvani, N. "Antibacterial Effect of the Culture Fluid of *Lentinus edodes* Mycelium Grown in Submerged Liquid Culture." *Int J Antimicrob Agents* 17:1 (2001): 71–74.

Hirasawa, M. "Three Kinds of Antibacterial Substances from *Lentinus edodes* (Berk.) Sing (Shiitake, an Edible Mushroom)." *Int J Antimicrob Agents* 11 (1999): 151–157.

Ikekawa, T., et al. "Anti-tumor Activity of Aqueous Extracts of Edible Mushrooms." *Cancer Res* 29 (1969): 734–735.

Kabir, Y., et al. "Dietary Mushrooms Reduce Blood Pressure in Spontaneously Hypertensive Rats." *J Nutr Sci Vitaminol* 35 (1989): 91–94.

Minato, K., et al. "Influence of Storage Conditions on Immunomodulating Activities of *Lentinus edodes*." *Int J Med Mushr* 1 (1999): 243–250.

Mizuno, T. "Bioactive Biomolecules of Mushrooms: Food Functions and Medicinal Effects of Mushroom Fungi." *Food Rev Intern* 11 (1995): 7–21.

Ng, M.L., et al.. "Inhibition of Human Colon Carcinoma Development by Lentinan from Shiitake Mushrooms (*Lentinula edodes*)." *J Altern Complement Med* 8:5 (2002): 581–589.

Ngai, P.H., et al. "Lentin, a Novel and Potent Antifungal Protein from Shiitake Mushroom with Inhibitory Effects on Activity of Human Immunodeficiency

Virus-1 Reverse Transcriptase and Proliferation of Leukemia Cells." *Life Sci* 73:26 (2003): 3363–3374.

Shouji, N. "Anticaries Effect of a Component from Shiitake (An Edible Mushroom)." *Caries Res* 34 (2000): 94–98.

Suzuki, H., et al. "Inhibition of the Infectivity and Cytopathologic Effect of Human Immunodeficiency Virus by Water-soluble Lignin in an Extract of the Culture Medium of *Lentinus edodes* Mycelia (LEM)." *Biochem Biophys Res Comm* 160 (1989): 367–373

Suzuki, S., et al. "Influence of Shiitake *Lentinus edodes* on Human Serum Cholesterol." *Annu Rep Natl Inst Nutr* 25 (1974): 89–94.

Yap, A.T., et al. "An Improved Method for the Isolation of Lentinan from the Edible and Medicinal Shiitake Mushroom, *Lentinus edodes* (Berk.) Sing. (Agaricomycetidae)." *Int J Med Mushr* 3 (2001): 6–19.

Zhu, X. "Treatment of Chronic Viral Hepatitis B and HBsAg Carriers with Polysaccharides of *Lentinus edodes*." *Jiangxi Zhongyiyao* 5 (1985): 20–25.

Chapter 6

El-Mekkawy, S., et al. "Anti-HIV-1 and anti-HIV-1-protease Substances from *Ganoderma lucidum*." *Phytochemistry* 49 (1998): 1651–1657.

Fujita, R., et al. "Anti-androgenic Activities of *Ganoderma lucidum*." *J Ethnopharmacol* (July 16, 2005).

Haijaj, H., et al. "Effect of 26-oxygeosterols from *Ganoderma lucidum* and their Activity as Cholesterol Synthesis Inhibitors." *Appl Environ Microbiol* 71:7 (2005): 3653–3658.

Hong, S.G., et al. "Phylogenetic Analysis of *Ganoderma* Based on Nearly Complete Mitochondrial Small-subunit Ribosomal DNA Sequences." *Mycologia* 96 (2004): 742–755.

Hsu, H.Y., et al. "Extract of Reishi Polysaccharides Induces Cytokine Expression via TLR4-modulated Protein Kinase Signaling Pathways." *J Immunol* 173:10 (2004): 5989–5999.

Iwatsuki, K., et al. "Lucidenic Acids P and Q, Methyl Lucidenate P, and Other Terpenoids from the Fungus *Ganoderma lucidum* and their Inhibitory Effects on Epstein-Barr Virus Activation." *J Natural Prod* 66:12 (2003): 1582–1585.

Jiang, J., et al. "*Ganoderma lucidum* Suppresses Growth of Breast Cancer Cells Through the Inhibition of Akt/NF-kappa Signaling." *Nutr Cancer* 49:2 (2004): 209–216.

Kim, K.C., et al. "*Ganoderma lucidum* Extracts Protect DNA from Strand Breakage Caused by Hydroxyl Radical and UV Irradiation." *Int J Mol Med* 4 (1999): 273–277.

Li, Z., et al. "Possible Mechanism Underlying the Antiherpetic Activity of a Proteoglycan Isolated from the Mycelia of *Ganoderma lucidum in vitro.*" *J Biochem Mol Biol* 38:1 (2005): 34–40.

Lin, S.B., et al. "Triterpene-enriched Extracts from *Ganoderma lucidum* Inhibit Growth of Hepatoma Cells via Suppressing Protein Kinase C, Activating Mitogen-activated Protein Kinases and G2-phase Cell Cycle Arrest." *Life Sci* 72:21 (2003): 2381–2390.

Lin, Z.B. "Focus on Anti-oxidative and Free Radical Scavenging Activity of *Ganoderma lucidum.*" *J Appl Pharmacol* 12 (2004): 133–137.

Lu, Q.Y., et al. "*Ganoderma lucidum* Extracts Inhibit Growth and Induce Actin Polymerization in Bladder Cancer Cells *in vitro.*" *Cancer Lett* 216:1 (2004): 9–20.

Lu, Q.Y., et al. "*Ganoderma lucidum* Spore Extract Inhibits Endothelial and Breast Cancer Cells *in vitro.*" *Oncol Rep* 12:3 (2004): 659–662.

Min, B.S., et al. "Triterpenes from the Spores of *Ganoderma lucidum* and their Cytotoxicity Against Meth-A and LLC Tumor Cells." *Chem Pharm Bull (Tokyo)* 48:7 (2000): 1026–1033.

Min, B.S., et al. "Anticomplement Activity of Terpenoids from the Spores of *Ganoderma lucidum.*" *Planta Med* 67 (2001): 811–814.

Moncalvo, J.M., et al. "Phylogenetic Relationships in *Ganoderma* Inferred from the Internal Transcribed Spacers and 25S Ribosomal DNA Sequences." *Mycologia* 87 (1995): 223–238.

Morigiwa, A., et al. "Angiotensin-converting Enzyme Inhibitory Triterpenes from *Ganoderma lucidum.*" *Chem Pharm Bull* 34 (1986): 3025–3028.

Mothama, R.A.A., et al. "Antiviral Lanostanoid Triterpenes from the Fungus *Ganoderma pfeifferi* BRES." *Fitoterapia* 74 (2003): 177–180.

Soo, T.S. "The Therapeutic Value of *Ganoderma lucidum.*" Abstract from the 8th International Mycological Congress, Vancouver, B.C., Canada, 1994.

Stanley, G., et al. "*Ganoderma lucidum* Suppresses Angiogenesis Through the Inhibition of Secretion of VEGF and TGF-beta1 from Prostate Cancer Cells." *Biochem Biophys Res Comm* 330:1 (2005): 46–52.

Su, C.Y., et al. "Predominant Inhibition of Ganodermic Acid S on the Thromboxane A2-dependent Pathway in Human Platelets Response to Collagen." *Biochim Biophys Acta* 1437 (1999): 223–234.

Wachtel-Galor, S., et al. "*Ganoderma lucidum* ("Lingzhi"), a Chinese Medicinal Mushroom: Biomarker Responses in a Controlled Human Supplementation Study." *Br J Nutr* 91:2 (2004): 171–173.

Wang, H., et al. "Ganodermin, an Antifungal Protein from Fruiting Bodies of the Medicinal Mushroom *Ganoderma lucidum.*" *Peptides* (July 20, 2005).

Wang, K.L., et al. "Antioxidant Activity of *Ganoderma lucidum* in Acute Ethanol-induced Heart Toxicity." *Phytother Res* 18:12 (2004): 1024–1026.

Wang, S.Y., et al. "The Anti-tumor *Ganoderma lucidum* is Mediated by Cytokines Released from Activated Macrophages and T Lymphocytes." *Int J Cancer* 70 (1997): 699–705.

Wasser, S.P. "Review of Medicinal Mushroom Advances: Good News from Old Allies." *HerbalGram* 56 (2002): 28–33.

Wen, M.C., et al. "Efficacy and Tolerability of Anti-asthma Herbal Medicine Intervention in Adult Patients with Moderate-severe Allergic Asthma." *J Allergy Clin Immunol* 116 (2005): 517–524.

Yan, R. "Treatment of Chronic Hepatitis B with Wulingdan Pill." *J 4th Milit Med Coll* 8 (1987): 380–383.

Yu, S., et al. "An Experimental Study on the Effects of Lingzhi Spore on the Immune Function and [60]Co Radioresistance in Mice." *J Natural Prod* 63:4 (2000): 514–516.

Zhang, H.N., et al. "Hypoglycemic Effect of *Ganoderma lucidum* Polysaccharides." *Acta Pharmacol Sin* 25:2 (2004): 191–195.

Zhu, M., et al. "Triterpene Antioxidants from *Ganoderma lucidum*." *Phytother Res* 13 (1999): 529–531.

Zhu, W.W., et al. "Effect of the Oil from *Ganoderma lucidum* Spores on Pathological Changes in the Substantia Nigra and Behaviors of MPTP-treated Mice." *Di Yi Jun Yi Da Xue Xue Bao* 25:6 (2005): 667–671.

Chapter 7

Bucci, L.R. "Selected Herbals and Human Exercise Performance." *Am J Clin Nutr* 72:2 Suppl (2000): 624S–636S.

Buchwald, D., et al. "Functional Status in Patients with Chronic Fatigue Syndrome, Other Fatiguing Illnesses, and Healthy Individuals." *Am J Med* 4 (1996): 364–370.

Cevallos-Casals, B.A., et al. "Stoichiometric and Kinetic Studies of Phenolic Antioxidants from Andean Purple Corn and Red-fleshed Sweet Potato." *J Agric Food Chem* 51:11 (2003): 3313–3319.

Che, Y.S., et al. "Observations on Therapeutic Effects of Jinshuibao on Coronary Heart Disease, Hyperlipidemia, and Blood Rheology." *Chin Trad Herb Dr* 9 (1996): 552–553.

Chen, D.G. "Effects of Jinshuibao Capsule on the Quality of Life of Patients with Heart Failure." *J Admin Trad Chin Med* 5 (1995): 40–43.

Clark, A.L., et al. "The Origin of Symptoms in Chronic Heart Failure." *Heart* 5 (1995): 429–430.

Crouse, S.F., et al. "Effects of Training and Single Session of Exercise on Lipids and Apolipoproteins in Hypercholesterolemic Men." *J Appl Physiol* 6 (1997): 2109–2028.

Fukuda, K., et al. "Chronic Fatigue Syndrome: A Comprehensive Approach to Its Definition and Study." *Ann Intern Med* (1994): 953–959.

Halpern, G.M. *Cordyceps: China's Healing Mushroom.* New York: Avery Publishing, 1998.

Holliday, J.C., et al. "Analysis of Quality and Techniques for Hybridization of Medicinal Fungus *Cordyceps sinensis* (Berk.) Sacc. (Ascomycetes)." *Int J Med Mushr* 6:2 (2004): 151–164.

Hsu, T.H., et al. "A Comparison of the Chemical Composition and Bioactive Ingredients of the Chinese Medicinal Mushroom DongChongXiaCao, Its Counterfeit and Mimic and Fermented Mycelium of *Cordyceps sinensis.*" *Food Chem* 78:4 (2002): 463–469.

Jones, K. "The Potential Health Benefits of Purple Corn." *HerbalGram* 85 (2005): 46–49.

Jiang, J.C., et al. "Summary of Treatment of 37 Chronic Renal Dysfunction Patients with Jinshuibao." *J Admin Trad Chin Med* 5 (1995): 23–24.

Kashyap, M.L. "Cholesterol and Atherosclerosis: A Contemporary Perspective." *Ann Acad Med Sin* 4 (1997): 517–523.

Kennedy H.L. "Beta Blockade, Ventricular Arrhythmias, and Sudden Cardiac Death." *Am J Card* 9b (1997): 29J–34J.

Kiho, T., et al. "Structural Features and Hypoglycemic Activity of a Polysaccharide (CS-F10) from the Cultured Mycelium of *Cordyceps sinensis.*" *Biol Pharm Bull* 22 (1999): 966–970.

Lei, M., et al. "Jinshubao Capsule as Adjuvant Treatment for Acute Stage Pulmonary Heart Disease: Analysis of Therapeutic Effect of 50 Clinical Cases." *J Admin Trad Chin Med* 5 (1995): 28–29.

Lemanske, R.E. "Asthma." *JAMA* 278 (1997): 1588–1593.

Lin, C.Y., et al. "Inhibition of Activated Human Mesangial Cell Proliferation by the Natural Product of *Cordyceps sinensis* (HY1-A): An Implication for Treatment of IgA Mesangial Nephropathy." *J Lab Clin Med* 33:1 (1999): 55–63.

Liu, C., et al. "Treatment of 22 Patients with Post-hepatitis Cirrhosis with a Preparation of Fermented Mycelia of *Cordyceps sinensis.*" *Shanghai J Chin Materia Med* 6 (1986): 30–31.

Manabe, N., et al. "Effects of the Mycelial Extract of Cultured *Cordyceps sinensis* on *in vivo* Hepatic Energy Metabolism in the Mouse." *Jpn J Pharmacol* 70:1 (1996): 85–88.

Manabe, N., et al. "Effects of the Mycelial Extract of Cultured *Cordyceps sinensis* on *in vivo* Hepatic Energy Metabolism and Blood Flow in Dietary Hypoferric Anaemic Mice." *Br J Nutr* 83:2 (2000): 197–204.

Markell, M.S. "Herbal Therapies and the Patient with Kidney Disease." *Qtr Rev Natural Med* Fall (1997): 189–200.

Pegler, D.N., et al. "The Chinese Caterpillar Fungus." *Mycologist* 8 (1994): 3–5.

Pereira, J. "Summer-plant-winter-worm." *NY J Med* 1 (1843): 128–132.

Shao, G., et al. "Treatment of Hyperlipidemia with *Cordyceps sinensis:* A Double-blind Placebo-control Trial." *Int Orient Med* 2 (1990): 77–80.

Siu, K.M., et al. "Pharmacological Basis of 'Yin-nourishing' and 'Yang-invigorating' Actions of *Cordyceps*, a Chinese Tonic Herb." *Life Sci* 76:4 (2004): 385–395.

Steinkraus, D.C., et al. "Chinese Caterpillar Fungus and World Record Runners." *Am Entomol* Winter (1994): 235–239.

Tsuda, T., et al. "Anthocyanin Enhances Adipocytokine Secretion and Adipocyte-specific Gene Expression in Isolated Rat Adipocytes." *Biochem Biophys Res Comm* 316 (2004): 149–157.

Uoma, P.V.I., et al. "High Serum Alpha-tocopherol, Albumin, Selenium, and Cholesterol, and Low Mortality from Coronary Disease in Northern Finland." *J Int Med* 237 (1995): 49–54.

Wang, Q., et al. "Comparison of Some Pharmacological Effects Between *Cordyceps sinensis* and *Cephalosporium sinensis*." *Bull Chin Materia Med* 12 (1987): 682–684.

Xie, F.Y. "Therapeutic Observation of Xingbao in Treating 83 Patients with Asymptomatic Hepatitis B." *Chin J Hosp Pharm* 8 (1992): 352–353.

Yamaguchi, N., et al. "Augmentation of Various Immune Reactivities of Tumor-bearing Hosts with an Extract of *Cordyceps sinensis*." *Biotherapy* 2:3 (1990): 199–205.

Zhang, C.K., et al. "Nourishment of *Cordyceps sinensis* Mycelium." *Weisheng-wuxue Tongbao* 19:3 (1992): 129–133.

Zhang, M., et al. "Notes on the Alpine *Cordyceps* of China and Nearby Nations." *Mycotaxon* 66 (1998): 215–229.

Zhang, Z., et al. "Clinical and Laboratory Studies of Jinshuibao in Scavenging Oxygen Free Radicals in Elderly Senescent Xuzheng Patients." *J Admin Trad Chin Med* 5 (1995): 14–18.

Zhao, C.S., et al. "CordyMax Cs-4 Improves Glucose Metabolism and Increases Insulin Sensitivity in Normal Rats." *J Altern Complement Med* 8:3 (2001): 309–314.

Zhu, J.S., G.M. Halpern, K. Jones. "The Scientific Rediscovery of an Ancient Chinese Herbal Medicine: *Cordyceps sinensis*." *J Altern Compl Med* 3 (1998): 239–303.

Chapter 8

Ellertsen, L.K., et al. "Effect of a Medicinal Extract from *Agaricus blazei* Murill on Gene Expression in Human Monocytes." Poster 1454, World Allergy Congress, Münich, Germany, June 26–30, 2005.

Fujimiya, Y., et al. "Selective Tumoricidal Effect of Soluble Proteoglucan Extracted from the Basidiomycete, *Agaricus blazei* Murill, Mediated via Natural Killer Cell Activation and Apoptosis." *Cancer Immunol Immunother* 46 (1998): 147–159.

Fujimiya, Y., et al. "Tumor-specific Cytocidal and Immunopotentiating Effects of Relatively Low Molecular Weight Products Derived from the Basidiomycete, *Agaricus blazei* Murill." *Anticancer Res* 19 (1999): 113–118.

Fujimiya, Y., et al. "Peroral Effect on Tumour Progression of Soluble Beta-(1,6)-glucans Prepared by Acid Treatment from *Agaricus blazei*. Murr. (Agaricaceae, Higher Basidiomycetes)." *Int J Med Mushr* 2 (2000): 43–49.

Ito, H., et al. "Anti-tumor Effects of a New Polysaccharide-protein Complex (ATOM) Prepared from *Agaricus blazei* (Iwade Strain 101) and Its Mechanisms in Tumor-bearing Mice." *Anticancer Res* 17 (1997): 277–284.

Kim, Y.W., et al. "Anti-diabetic Activity of Beta-glucans and Their Enzymatically Hydrolyzed Oligosaccharides from *Agaricus blazei*." *Biotechnol Lett* 27:7 (2005): 483–487.

Kimura, Y., et al. "Isolation of an Anti-angiogenic Substance from *Agaricus blazei* Murrill: Its Antitumor and Antimetastatic Actions." *Cancer Sci* 95:9 (2004): 758–764.

Mizuno, T., et al. "Antitumor Activity and Some Properties of Water-soluble Polysaccharides from "Himematsutake," the Fruiting Body of *Agaricus blazei* Murrill." *Agr Biol Chem (Tokyo)* 54 (1990): 2889–2896.

Mizuno, M., et al. "Polysaccharides from *Agaricus blazei* Stimulate Lymphocyte T-cell Subsets in Mice." *Biosci Biotechnol Biochem* 62 (1998): 434–437.

Mizuno, T., et al. "Anti-tumor Polysaccharide from the Mycelium of Liquid-cultured *Agaricus blazei* Mill." *Biochem Mol Biol Int* 47:4 (1999): 707–714.

Ohno, N., et al. "Antitumor Beta-glucan from the Cultured Fruit-body of *Agaricus blazei*." *Biol Pharm Bull* 24:7 (2001): 820–828.

Stijve, T., et al. "*Agaricus blazei* Murrill—A New Gourmet and Medicinal Mushroom From Brazil." *Australasian Mycologist* 21:1 (2002): 29–33.

Takaku, T., et al. "Isolation of an Antitumor Compound from *Agaricus blazei* Murrill and Its Mechanism of Action." *J Nutr* 131:5 (2001): 1409–1413.

Wasser, S.P., et al. "Is a Widely Cultivated Culinary-medicinal Royal Sun *Agaricus* (The Himematsutake Mushroom) Indeed *Agaricus blazei* Murrill?" *Int J Med Mushr* 4 (2002): 267–290.

Chapter 9

DPRKorea-Trade. "Phellinus linteus—The Elexir for Health and Long Life." Available online at: http://www.dprkorea-trade.com/sang/sang01.htm.

Han, S.B., et al. "The Inhibitory Effect of Polysaccharides Isolated from *Phellinus linteus* on Tumor Growth and Metastasis." *Immunopharmacol* 42 (1999): 157–164.

Hur, J.M., et al. "Antibacterial Effect of *Phellinus linteus* Against Methicillin-resistant *Staphylococcus aureus*." *Fitoterapia* 75:6 (2004): 603–605.

Kim, H.M., et al. "Stimulation of Humoral and Cell-mediated Immunity by Polysaccharide from Mushroom *Phellinus linteus*." *Int J Immunopharmacol* 18 (1996): 295–303.

Kim, S.H., et al. "Anti-inflammatory and Related Pharmacological Activities of the n-BuOH Subfraction of Mushroom *Phellinus linteus*." *J Ethnopharmacol* 93:1 (2004): 141–146.

Lim, B.O., et al. "Comparative Study on the Modulation of IgE and Cytokine Production by *Phellinus linteus* Grown on Germinated Brown Rice, *Phellinus linteus* and Germinated Brown Rice in Murine Splenocytes." *Biosci Biotechnol Biochem* 68:11 (2004): 2391–2394.

Shibata, Y., et al. "Dramatic Remission of Hormone Refractory Prostate Cancer Achieved with Extract of the Mushroom, *Phellinus linteus*." *Urol Int* 73:2 (2004): 188–190.

Ying, J., et al. *Icones of Medicinal Fungi from China.* Beijing, China: Science Press, 1987.

Chapter 10

Cancer Research UK. "Medicinal Mushrooms and Cancer." Available online at: http://www.sci.cancerresearchuk.org/labs/med_mush/med_mush.html.

Dong, Y., et al. "*In vitro* Inhibition of Proliferation of HL-60 Cells by Tetrandrine and Peptides Derived from Chinese Medicinal Herbs." *Life Sci* 60 (1997): 135–140.

Fujimoto, S., et al. "Clinical Value of Immunochemotherapy with OK-432." *Jpn J Surg* 3 (1979): 190–196.

Hayakawa, K., et al. "Effect of Krestin (PSK) as Adjuvant Treatment on the Prognosis after Radical Radiotherapy in Patients with Non-small Cell Lung Cancer." *Anticancer Res* 13 (1993): 1815–1820.

Ikusawa, T., et al. "Fate and Distribution of an Anti-tumour Protein-bound Polysaccharide PSK (Krestin)." *Int J Immunopharmacol* 10 (1988): 415–423.

Jian, Z.H., et al. "The Effect of PSP and LAK Cell Function." In Yang, Q.Y. (ed.).

Advanced Research in PSP. Hong Kong: Hong Kong Association for Health Care, 1999, pp. 143–150.

Jong, S., et al. "PSP—A Powerful Biological Response Modifier from the Mushroom *Coriolus versicolor.*" In Yang, Q.Y. (ed.). *Advanced Research in PSP.* Hong Kong: Hong Kong Association for Health Care, 1999, pp. 16–18.

Kaibarara, N., et al. "Postoperative Long-term Chemotherapy for Advanced Gastric Cancer." *Jpn J Surg* 6 (1976): 54–59.

Kidd, P.M. "The Use of Mushroom Glucans and Proteoglycans in Cancer Therapy." *Altern Med Rev* 5 (2000): 4–27.

Koch, J., et al. "The Influence of Selected Basidiomycetes on the Binding of Lipopolysaccharide to Its Receptor." *Int J Med Mush* 4 (2002): 229–235.

Kondo, M., et al. "Evaluation of an Anticancer Activity of a Protein-bound Polysaccharide PSK (Krestin)." In Torisu, M., and T. Yoshida (eds.). *Basic Mechanisms and Clinical Treatment of Tumour Metastasis.* New York: Academic Press, 1985, pp. 623–636.

Lau, C.B., et al. "Cytotoxic Activities of *Coriolus versicolor* (Yungzhi) Extract on Human Leukemia and Lymphoma Cells by Induction of Apoptosis." *Life Sci* 75:7 (2004): 797–808.

Lino, Y., et al. "Immunochemotherapies vs. Chemotherapy as Adjuvant Treatment after Curative Resection of Operable Breast Cancer." *Anticancer Res* 15 (1995): 2907–2912.

Liu, F., et al. "Induction in the Mouse of Gene Expression of Immunomodulating Cytokines by Mushroom Polysaccharide Complexes." *Life Sci* 58 (1996): 1795–1803.

Liu, J.X., et al. "Phase II Clinical Trial for PSP Capsules." *PSP International Symposium.* Shanghai, China: Fudan University Press, 1993.

Liu, J.X., et al. "Phase III Clinical Trial for Yun Zhi Polysaccharopeptide (PSP) Capsules." In Yang, Q.Y. (ed.). *Advanced Research in PSP.* Hong Kong: Hong Kong Association for Health Care, 1999, pp. 295–303.

Liu, L.F. "PSP in Clinical Cancer Therapy." In Yang, Q.Y. (ed.). *Advanced Research in PSP.* Hong Kong: Hong Kong Association for Health Care, 1999, pp. 68–75.

Mao, X.W., et al. "Effects of Extract of *Coriolus versicolor* and IL-2 on Radiation Against Three Tumor Lines." Lorna Linda University, unpublished data, 1998.

McCune, C.S., et al. "Basic Concepts of Tumour Immunology and Principles of Immunotherapy." In *Clinical Oncology,* 7th edition. Philadelphia: W.B. Saunders, 1993, p. 123.

Morimoto, T., et al. "Postoperative Adjuvant Randomised Trial Comparing Chemoendocrine Therapy, Chemotherapy and Immunotherapy for Patients with Stage II Breast Cancer: 5-year Results from the Nishimihou Cooperative Study

Group of Adjuvant Chemoendocrine Therapy for Breast Cancer (ACETBC) of Japan." *Eur J Cancer* 32A (1996): 235–242.

Nakazato, H., et al. "Efficacy of Immunochemotherapy as Adjuvant Treatment after Curative Resection of Gastric Cancer." *Lancet* 343 (1994): 1122–1126.

Ng, T.B., et al. "Polysaccharopeptide from the Mushroom *Coriolus versicolor* Possesses Analgesic Activity but Does Not Produce Adverse Effects on Female Reproduction or Embryonic Development in Mice." *Gen Pharmacol* 29 (1997): 269–273.

Ogoshi, K., et al. "Possible Predictive Markers of Immunotherapy in Oesophageal Cancer: Retrospective Analysis of a Randomised Study." *Cancer Investig* 13 (1995): 363–369.

Okazaki, M., et al. "Structure-activity Relationship of (1-3)-(-D-glucan in the Induction of Cytokine Production from Macrophages *in vitro*." *Biol Pharmacol Bull* 18 (1995): 1320–1327.

Qian, Z.M., et al. "Polysaccharide Peptide (PSP) Restores Immunosuppression Induced by Cyclophosphamide." In Yang, Q.Y. (ed.). *Advanced Research in PSP*. Hong Kong: Hong Kong Association for Health Care, 1999, pp. 154–163.

Sakagami, H., et al. "Induction of Immunopotentiation Activity by a Protein-bound Polysaccharide, PSK." *Anticancer Res* 11 (1991): 993–1000.

Shiu, W.C.T., et al. "A Clinical Study of PSP on Peripheral Blood Counts During Chemotherapy." *Physiol Res* 6 (1992): 217–218.

Stephens, L.C., et al. "Apoptosis in Irradiated Murine Tumours." *Radiation Res* 127 (1991): 308.

Sugimachi, K., et al. "Hormone Conditional Cancer Chemotherapy for Recurrent Breast Cancer Prolongs Survival." *Jpn J Surg* 14 (1994): 217–221.

Sun, Z., et al. "The Ameliorative Effect of PSP on the Toxic and Side Reaction of Chemo- and Radiotherapy of Cancers." In Yang, Q.Y. (ed.). *Advanced Research in PSP.* Hong Kong: Hong Kong Association for Health Care, 1999.

Toi, M., et al. "Randomised Adjuvant Trial to Evaluate the Addition of Tamoxifen and PSK to Chemotherapy in Patients with Primary Breast Cancer." *Cancer* 70 (1992): 2475–2483.

Tochikura, T.S., et al. "A Biological Response Modifier, PSK, Inhibits Human Immunodeficiency Virus Infection *in vitro*." *Biochem Biophys Res Comm* 148 (1987): 726–733.

Tsang, K.W., et al. "*Coriolus versicolor* Polysaccharide Peptide Slows Progression of Advanced Non-small Cell Lung Cancer." *Resp Med* 97:6 (2003): 618–624.

Tsujitani, S., et al. "Postoperative Adjuvant Immunochemotherapy and Infiltration of Dendritic Cells for Patients with Advanced Gastric Cancer." *Anticancer Res* 12 (1992): 645–648.

Chapter 177

Tsukagoshi, S., et al. "Krestin (PSK)." *Cancer Treat Rev* 11 (1984): 131–155.

Tzianabos; A. "Polysaccharide Immunomodulators as Therapeutic Agents: Structural Aspects and Biologic Functions." *Clin Microbiol Rev* 13 (2000): 523–533.

Yang, Q.Y. (ed.). *Advanced Research in PSP.* Hong Kong: Hong Kong Association for Health Care, 1999.

Yao, W. "Prospective Randomised Trial of Radiotherapy Plus PSP in the Treatment of Oesophageal Carcinoma." In Yang, Q.Y. (ed.). *Advanced Research in PSP.* Hong Kong: Hong Kong Association for Health Care, 1999, pp. 310–313.

Yokoe, T., et al. "HLA Antigen as Predictive Index for the Outcome of Breast Cancer Patients with Adjuvant Immunochemotherapy with PSK." *Anticancer Res* 17 (1997): 2815–2818.

Zhong, B.Z., et al. "Genetic Toxicity Test of Yun Zhi Polysaccharide (PSP)." In Yang, Q.Y. (ed.). *Advanced Research in PSP.* Hong Kong: Hong Kong Association for Health Care, 1999, pp. 285–294.

Chapter 11

Ito, M., et al. "Anti-tumor Activity of Hot-water Extract of *Hericium erinaceus* (Yamabushitake)." *Nature Med* 53 (1999): 263–265.

Kenmoku, H., et al. "Erinacine Q, A New Erinacine From *Hericium erinaceum* and Its Biosynthetic Route to Erinacine C in the Basidiomycete." *Biosci Biotechnol Biochem* 66 (2002): 571–575.

Mizuno, T. "Yamabushitake. *Hericium erinaceum:* Bioactive Substances and Medical Utilization." *Food Rev Intl* 11 (1995): 173–178.

Mizuno, T. "Bioactive Substances in *Hericium erinaceus* (Bull.: fr) pers. (Yamabushitake), and Its Medicinal Utilization." *Int J Med Mushr* 1 (1999): 105–119.

Saito, T., et al. "Erinacine E as a Kappa Opioid Receptor Agonist and Its New Analogs From a Basidiomycete, *Hericium ramosum.*" *J Antibiot* 51 (1998): 983–990.

Wang, J.C., et al. "Antitumor and Immunoenhancing Activities of Polysaccharide from Culture Broth of *Hericium* spp." *Kaohsiung J Med Sci* 17:9 (2001): 461–467.

Wang, J.C., et al. "Hypoglycemic Effect of Extract of *Hericium erinaceus.*" *J Sci Food Agric* 85:4 (2005): 641–646.

Yang, B.K., et al. "Hypolipidemic Effect of an Exo-biopolymer Produced from a Submerged Mycelial Culture of *Hericium erinaceus.*" *Biosci Biotechnol Biochem* 67:6 (2003): 1292–1298.

Xu, H.M., et al. "Immunomodulatory Function of Polysaccharide of *Hericium erinaceus.*" *Chung kuo chung his I chieh ho tsa chih* 14 (1994): 427–428.

Chapter 12

Batterbury, M., et al. "*Agaricus bisporus* (Edible Mushroom Lectin) Inhibits Ocular Fibroblast Proliferation and Collagen Lattice Contraction." *Exp Eye Res* 74:3 (2002): 361–370.

Carrizo, M.E., et al. "The Antineoplastic Lectin of the Common Edible Mushroom (*Agaricus bisporus*) has Two Binding Sites, Each Specific for a Different Configuration at a Single Epimeric Hydroxyl." *J Biol Chem* 280:11 (2005): 10614–10623.

Chen, et al. "Neuroprotective Diterpenes from the Fruiting Body of *Antrodia camphorata*." *J Nat Prod* 69:4 (2006): 689–691.

Cheng, J.J., et al. "Characterization and Functional Study of *Antrodia camphorata* Lipopolysaccharide." *J Agric Food Chem* 53:2 (2005): 469–474.

Gao, Q.P., et al. "Characterization and Cytokine Stimulating Activities of Heteroglycans from *Tremella fuciformis*." *Planta Med* 62:4 (1996): 297–302.

Grube, B.J., et al. "White Button Mushroom Phytochemicals Inhibit Aromatase Activity and Breast Cancer Cell Proliferation." *J Nutr* 131:12 (2001): 3288–3293.

Hara, C., et al. "Anti-inflammatory Activity and Conformational Behavior of a Branched (1 leads to 3)-Beta-D-glucan from an Alkaline Extract of *Dictyophora indusiata* Fisch." *Carbohydr Res* 110:1 (1982): 77–87.

Hseu, Y.C., et al. "Anti-inflammatory Potential of *Antrodia camphorata* Through Inhibition of iNOS, COX-2 and Cytokines via the NF-kappa B Pathway." *Int Immunopharmacol* 5:13–14 (2005): 1914–1925.

Hseu, Y.C., et al. "Induction of Apoptosis by *Antrodia camphorata* in Human Premyelocytic Leukemia HL-60 Cells." *Nutr Cancer* 48:2 (2004): 189–197.

Hsiao, G., et al. "Antioxidative and Hepatoprotective Effects of *Antrodia camphorata* Extract." *J Agric Food Chem* 51:11 (2003): 3302–3308.

Kawagishi, H., et al. "Dictyophorines A and B, Two Stimulators of NGF-Synthesis from the Mushroom *Dictyophora indusiata*." *Phytochemistry* 45:6 (1997): 1203–1205.

Kent, D., et al. "Edible Mushroom (*Agaricus bisporus*) Lectin Inhibits Human Retinal Pigment Epithelial Cell Proliferation *in Vitro*." *Wound Repair Regen* 11:4 (2003): 285–291.

Kent, D., et al. "Edible Mushroom (*Agaricus bisporus*) Lectin Modulates Human Retinal Pigment Epithelial Cell Behaviour *in Vitro*." *Exp Eye Res* 76:2 (2003): 213–219.

Kiho, T., et al. "Polysaccharides in Fungi. XXXIII. Hypoglycemic Activity of an Acidic Polysaccharide (AC) from *Tremella fuciformis*." (Article in Japanese.) *Yakugaku Zasshi* 114:5 (1994): 308–315.

Chapter 179

Lee, I.K., et al. "Dictyoquinazols A, B, and C, New Neuroprotective Compounds from the Mushroom *Dictyophora indusiata*." *J Nat Prod* 65:12 (2002): 1769–1772.

Li, G.H., et al. "Nematicidal Activity and Chemical Component of *Poria cocos*." *J Microbiol* 43:1 (2005): 17–20.

Lin, W.C., et al. "Filtrate of Fermented Mycelia from *Antrodia camphorata* Reduces Liver Fibrosis Induced by Carbon Tetrachloride in Rats." *World J Gastroenterol* 12:15 (2006): 2369–2374.

Piraino, F., and C.R. Brandt. "Isolation and Partial Characterization of an Antiviral, RC-183, from the Edible Mushroom *Rozites caperata*." *Antiviral Res* 43:2 (1999): 67–78.

Reshetnikov, S.V., et al. "Medicinal Value of the Genus *Tremella* Pers. (Heterobasidiomycetes)." (Review). *Int J Med Mushrooms* 2 (2000): 345–367.

Stamets, Paul. "Antipox Properties of *Fomitopsis officinalis* (Vill.: Fr.) Bond. et Singer (Agarikon) from the Pacific Northwest of North America." *Int J Med Mush* 7:3 (2005): 213.

Volk, Tom. Tom Volk's Fungi. Available online at: http://TomVolkFungi.net.

Volk, Tom. "*Tremella fuciformis*, the Snow Fungus, an Edible Jelly Fungus." Available online at: http://botit.botany.wisc.edu/toms_fungi/jan2006.html.

Volk, Tom. "Tom Volk's Fungus of the Month for November 1999." Available online at: http://botit.botany.wisc.edu/toms_fungi/nov99.html.

Wu, S.-H., L. Ryvarden, and T.-T. Chang. "*Antrodia camphorata* ("niu-chang-chih"), New Combination of a Medicinal Fungus in Taiwan." *Bot Bull Acad Sin* 38 (1997): 273–275. Available online at: http://ejournal.sinica.edu.tw/bbas/content/1997/4/bot384-09.pdf.

Yang, H.L., et al. "Growth Inhibition and Induction of Apoptosis in MCF-7 Breast Cancer Cells by *Antrodia camphorata*." *Cancer Lett* 231:2 (2006): 215–227.

Zhang, G.W., et al. "Anti-rejection Effect of Ethanol Extract of *Poria cocos* Wolf in Rats After Cardiac Allograft Implantation." *Chin Med J (Engl)* 117:6 (2004): 932–935.

Chapter 13

Cancer Research UK. "Medicinal Mushrooms and Cancer." Available online at: http://www.sci.cancerresearchuk.org/labs/med_mush/med_mush.html.

Glasser, V. "Billion Dollar Market Blossoms as Botanicals Take Root." *Nature Biotech* 17 (1999): 17–18.

Huxtable, R.H. "The Safety of Botanicals: A Historical Perspective." In Eshkimazi, D. (ed.). *Botanical Medicine*. Larchmont, NY: Mary-Ann Liebert, 1999, pp. 87–101.

Kabir, Y., et al. "Dietary Mushrooms Reduce Blood Pressure in Spontaneously Hypertensive Rats (SHR)." *J Nutr Sci Vitaminol (Tokyo)* 35 (1989): 91–94.

Pezzuto, J.H. "Plant-derived Anticancer Agents." *Biochem Pharmacol* 53 (1997): 121–133.

Raverat, Gwen. *Period Piece.* East Lansing, MI: University of Michigan Press, 1991.

Sawai, M., et al. "Extraction of Conformationally Stable (1-6)-branched (1-3)-(-glucans from Premixed Edible Mushroom Powders by Cold-alkaline Solution." *Int J Med Mushr* 4 (2002): 3.

Wang, R.W., et al. "Clinical Trial of *Immune-Assist:* A Mixture of Six Medicinal Mushroom Extracts for Cancer Treatment." *Int J Med Mushr* (In press).

Wasser, S.P., et al. "Dietary Supplements from Medicinal Mushrooms: Diversity of Types and Variety of Regulations." *Int J Med Mushr* 2 (2000): 1–20.

Wasser, S.P., et al. "The Regulation of Dietary Supplements from Medicinal Mushrooms." In Van Griensven (ed.). *Science and Cultivation of Edible Fungi.* Rotterdam: Balkeina, 2000, pp. 789–801.

Wasser, S.P. "Review of Medicinal Mushroom Advances: Good News from Old Allies." *HerbalGram* 56 (2002): 28–33.

Wedam, W., et al. "Breast Cancer." *J Naturopath Med* 7 (1997): 86–87.

Zhu, J., et al. "Amphiphilic Core-shell Nanoparticles with Poly(ethylenimine) Shells as Potential Gene Delivery Carriers." *Bioconjug Chem* 16:1 (2005): 139–146.

Index